35

What's Wrong
with
My Gallbladder?
Understanding Laparoscopic
Cholecystectomy

What's Wrong
with
My Gallbladder?
Understanding Laparoscopic Cholecystectomy

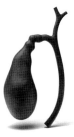

Wei-Liang Loh
Singapore Health Services, Singapore

Konrad Ong
University of Queensland, Australia

Natalie Ngoi
National University Health System, Singapore

Sing Shang Ngoi
NUS, Singapore & Ngoi Surgery Pte. Ltd, Singapore

World Scientific

NEW JERSEY · LONDON · SINGAPORE · BEIJING · SHANGHAI · HONG KONG · TAIPEI · CHENNAI · TOKYO

Published by

World Scientific Publishing Co. Pte. Ltd.

5 Toh Tuck Link, Singapore 596224

USA office: 27 Warren Street, Suite 401-402, Hackensack, NJ 07601

UK office: 57 Shelton Street, Covent Garden, London WC2H 9HE

Library of Congress Cataloging-in-Publication Data
Loh, Wei-Liang.
    What's wrong with my gallbladder? : understanding laparoscopic cholecystectomy /
Wei-Liang Loh, Singapore Health Services, Singapore, [and three others].
      pages cm
    Includes bibliographical references and index.
      ISBN 978-9814723497 (hardcover : alk. paper) -- ISBN 978-9814723503 (pbk. : alk. paper)
    1. Gallbladder--Surgery. 2. Laparoscopic surgery. 3. Cholecystectomy. I. Title.
    RD546.L596 2016
    617.5'565--dc23

                                                            2015034545

British Library Cataloguing-in-Publication Data
A catalogue record for this book is available from the British Library.

Typeset by Stallion Press
Email: enquiries@stallionpress.com

Printed in Singapore

Contents

Introduction	1
Basic Relevant Anatomy and Physiology	3
Indications and Contraindications	11
Diagnosis	35
Pre-operative Assessment	51
Operative Procedure	55
Post-operative Phase	87
Complications	91
3D Laparoscopic Surgery for Cholecystectomy	103
Single Incision Laparoscopic Surgery for Cholecystectomy	107
Robotic Surgery for Cholecystectomy	115
Challenging Scenarios	117
Frequently Asked Questions	135
Conclusion	143
Appendix: Equipment	145
Index	171

Introduction

The word laparoscopy comes from the ancient Greek word of *lapara*, meaning "flank" or "side", and *skopeó*, meaning "to see". Cholecystectomy means the surgical removal of the gallbladder, originating from the Ancient Greek words *cholé* and *kystis* — which mean "bile" and "bladder" respectively. Put together, laparoscopic cholecystectomy means the surgical removal of the gallbladder via small incisions on the abdomen to permit entry of a camera and customized instruments.

Laparoscopic surgery first found favour among gynaecologists for removal of tumours and other masses from the female genitourinary tract. The first laparoscopic cholecystectomy was performed in the 1980's. It met with some initial resistance from general surgeons, who belittled the revolutionary technique as a gimmick. However, it was not long before the safety, and the significant reduction in post-operative recovery period and pain of the new technique resulted in widespread acceptance amongst general surgeons. Laparoscopic cholecystectomy is now the established procedure of choice for routine removal of the gallbladder for symptomatic cholelithiasis (or gallstones), and is the most widely performed elective general surgical operation currently.

The use of laparoscopy has become widespread and recognised as the standard of care in a myriad of general surgical, gynaecological and urological procedures. The use of endoscopes has also spread to surgical specialties such as otorhinolaryngology, thoracic surgery, orthopaedic surgery and neurosurgery.

Indeed, endoscopic surgery is here to stay and better accessories are being produced to maximise a surgeon's performance. These include high-definition camera systems (including 3-dimensional systems), cutting-edge energy devices, more ergonomically made instruments and the use of robotic systems.

This book serves primarily to bridge the knowledge gap between surgeons and their patients by explaining in detail the various aspects of this common procedure. This book has been written intentionally with a more technical slant, especially for the chapter on operative procedures (Operative Procedure, page 55), so as to allow its readers to be conversant in the finer details of the procedure. As such, this book is highly recommended for medical students and junior surgical trainees interested in the intricacies of laparoscopic cholecystectomy, and in acquiring the technical know-how to perform it in a safe and technically-sound manner. It is also hoped that patients undergoing this procedure and their concerned relatives can use this book to answer any questions that they may have about the procedure, as well as to allay their fears.

Basic Relevant Anatomy and Physiology

Anatomy

The bile ducts begin primarily as bile canaliculi in the parenchyma of the liver as part of the portal triad. The canaliculi join to form progressively larger biliary radicals, with each liver segment having its own biliary branch. These branches ultimately form the extra-hepatic left and right hepatic ducts. The hepatic ducts join at the porta hepatis to form the common hepatic duct, which then begins its descent within the hepatoduodenal ligament in unison with the portal vein and proper hepatic artery. The portal vein lies posterior to both the hepatic duct and hepatic artery, with the duct usually to the right of the artery.

The common hepatic duct becomes the common bile duct at the junction where the cystic duct from the gallbladder joins it. It then continues to the ampulla of Vater where it is joined by the main pancreatic duct, emptying into the medial wall of the second part of the duodenum (Figs. 1 and 2). The sphincter of Oddi marks the entrance of the biliopancreatic tree into the duodenum.

The gallbladder is a pear-shaped organ lying below segments 4 and 5 of the liver inferiorly. Its normal size ranges from 5–10 cm in length, and 3–6 cm in diameter. It normally stores up to 60 ml of fluid, but its capacity can increase dramatically under certain pathological conditions that cause the accumulation of bile.

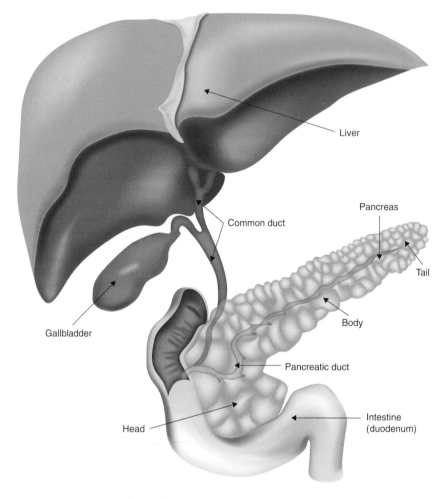

Figure 1.   Relation of common bile duct to the pancreas and its duct.

The gallbladder is split into four different parts for ease of description: the fundus, body, infundibulum and neck. Hartmann's pouch is an out-pouching of the gallbladder at the region of the neck formed secondary to an obstruction at the cystic duct, and its size can vary greatly due to the degree of obstruction (Fig. 3). The neck of the gallbladder leads to the cystic duct, which forms the main connection of the gallbladder to the rest of the

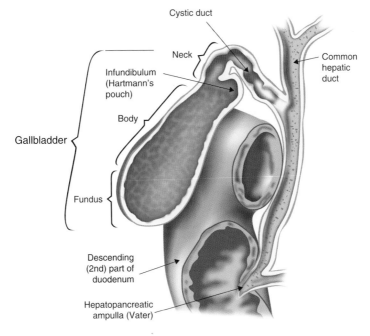

Figure 2.   Normal gallbladder anatomy in relation to adjacent structures.

extra-hepatic biliary tree for the flow of bile. Accessory ducts of Luschka connect the hepatic parenchyma directly to the gallbladder as well. The cystic duct ranges from 1–5 cm in length depending on the level at which it joins the extra-hepatic biliary tree, and is usually 3–8 mm in width. Within the cystic duct are spiral valves that help to regulate the flow of bile to and from the gallbladder. There are many variants of cystic duct anatomy in terms of its position and entry into the common bile duct, which the surgeon must be aware of in order to avoid injury to the extra-hepatic biliary tree (Fig. 4).

The blood supply to the gallbladder is highly fickle, but is usually supplied by a single cystic artery, arising most commonly from the right hepatic artery. Variants include the cystic artery coming off the left hepatic, gastroduodenal or superior mesenteric arteries. A double cystic artery may be present, and small branches from the liver provide additional blood supply to the gallbladder (Fig. 5).

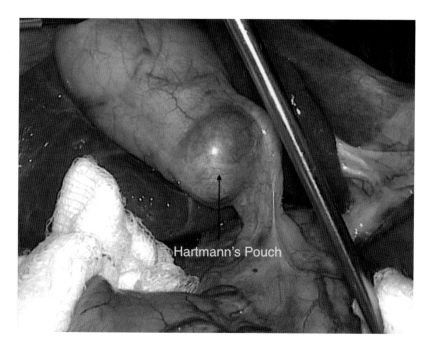
Hartmann's Pouch

Figure 3.   Intra-operative visualization of Hartmann's pouch before dissection begins.

Calot's triangle is one of the most critical anatomical landmarks with regards to cholecystectomy, and its visualisation carries great importance in the avoidance of incidental injury to the biliary tree. It is bound by the common hepatic duct medially, the inferior edge of the liver superiorly, and the cystic duct laterally. The cystic artery is usually found within this triangle, after it has branched off from the right hepatic artery. The presence of the lymph node of Cloquet accurately predicts the location of the cystic artery, and is the main route of lymphatic drainage (Figs. 6 and 7).

Physiology

The liver produces bile continuously, and its transport is via the bile canaliculi, which flows progressively into larger biliary channels. The daily production of bile ranges from 500 ml to 1000 ml. Bile is composed mainly of water, electrolytes, bile salts, proteins, lipids and bile pigments.

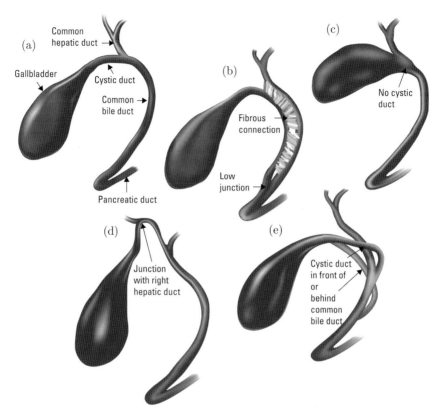

Figure 4. Common variants of cystic duct anatomy.

The primary bile salts cholate and chenodeoxycholate are synthesized from cholesterol in the liver, following which they undergo conjugation with the amino acids glycine and taurine. The conjugated bile salts are then excreted into bile by hepatocytes. The majority of bile is stored in the gallbladder during fasting. Following a meal, the gastrointestinal hormone cholecystokinin causes the contraction of the gallbladder with the subsequent emptying of 50–70% of its contents into the duodenum via the common bile duct.

Bile salts mixes with ingested food in the small intestines and aids in the absorption and digestion of fats. Ninety-five percent of the bile acid pool is reabsorbed and returned to the liver via the portal venous system, otherwise

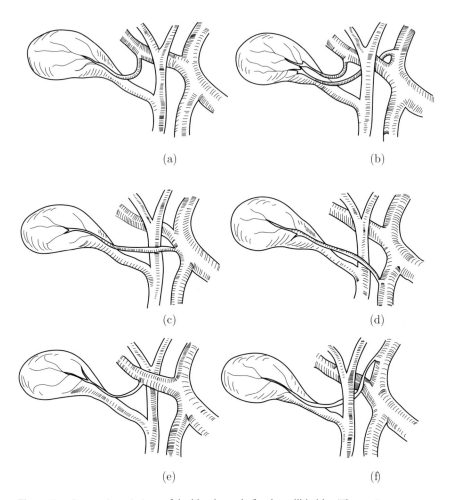

Figure 5.   Anatomic variations of the blood supply for the gallbladder. The cystic artery usually arises from the right hepatic artery (a). Variations to this usual anatomy include dual cystic arteries, one arising from each of the hepatic arteries (b); cystic artery arising from the common hepatic artery (c); cystic artery arising from the gastroduodenal artery (d); cystic artery arising from an anterior right hepatic artery (e); a single cystic artery arising from the left hepatic artery (f).

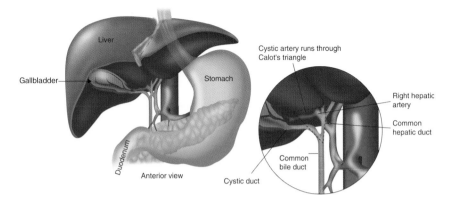

Figure 6. Importance of Calot's triangle in identifying the cystic artery.

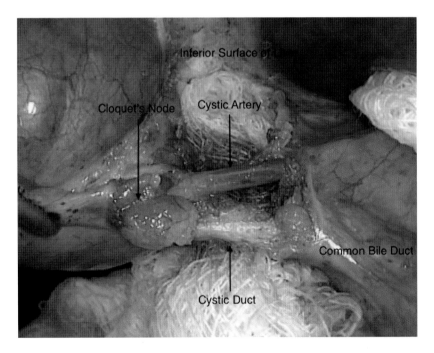

Figure 7. Calot's triangle dissected with cystic artery identified within.

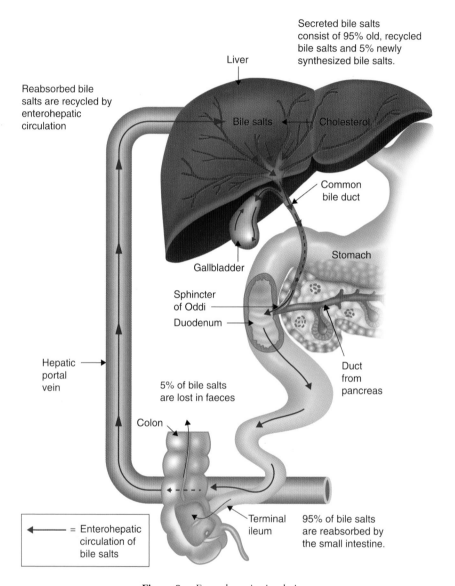

Figure 8. Enterohepatic circulation.

Indications and Contraindications

Gallstones and the myriad of pathological conditions it causes are by far the most common reason cholecystectomies are carried out. Broadly speaking, there are three main types of gallstones: (1) calcium, bilirubin and pigmented; (2) cholesterol; and (3) mixed types.

Formation of Gallstones

Under physiological conditions, bile is made up of a mixture of water, bile salts, mucus, bile pigments, cholesterol and inorganic salts. It is kept in solution by a delicate balance of each of its individual components. Pathological processes, which tilt one constituent too far in either direction, may allow precipitation of the various components of bile. Microscopic crystals are first formed from the precipitation, whence they get trapped in gallbladder mucus to form gallbladder sludge. As the conditions that enable precipitation continue, the crystals increase in number, aggregate and combine to form macroscopic stones.

They most commonly form in the gallbladder, but similar biochemical derangements can also cause stones to form in the bile ducts (including the common bile duct, common hepatic duct, right and left hepatic ducts, and even the smaller biliary ducts) themselves, whereby they are known as primary ductal stones.

Calcium, Bilirubin and Pigmented Gallstones

Calcium is an inorganic ion that enters bile in the same passive manner as other electrolytes. Bilirubin is a yellow pigment resulting from the breakdown of heme, and is actively secreted by liver parenchymal cells into bile. The majority of bilirubin is in the form of glucuronide conjugates that are water soluble, but a small fraction exists as unconjugated bilirubin that tends to form insoluble precipitates with calcium.

Unconjugated bilirubin may be present in concentrations higher than normal in conditions that lead to excess heme turnover. The calcium ions may precipitate with the excess unconjugated bilirubin to form calcium bilirubinate. Different oxidative reactions cause the bilirubin precipitates to turn black, hence the term black pigment gallstones (Fig. 1). Their presence at an early age may be indicative of a pathological process resulting in excess haemolysis and increased bilirubin secretion into bile, including conditions such as thalassemia, hereditary spherocytosis or sickle cell anaemia. Patients with cirrhosis are also predisposed to pigment gallstone formation; this occurs as portal hypertension-induced splenomegaly causes red blood cell sequestration, with a subsequent increase in heme turnover.

Black pigment stones may also form in situations where normally sterile bile becomes colonised with bacteria. This may occur upstream to a biliary stricture causing bile stasis. The bacteria then hydrolyse the water-soluble conjugated bilirubin into unconjugated bilirubin, and precipitation of calcium bilirubinate may ensue. Such strictures are commonly due to choledochal cysts, post-surgical biliary strictures, malignancy or inflammatory conditions of the biliary tract.

The presence of bacteria also hydrolyses lecithin contained within bile to release fatty acids, which are also capable of precipitating with calcium. They result in a brown, claylike coalescence and are termed brown pigment stones. These stones usually form within the extrahepatic and intrahepatic bile ducts as a result of liver fluke infestation, and are known as hepatolithiasis.

Cholesterol Gallstones

Cholesterol gallstones are made up of 80% or more cholesterol by weight, and their appearance can vary from light yellow to dark green or brown, and

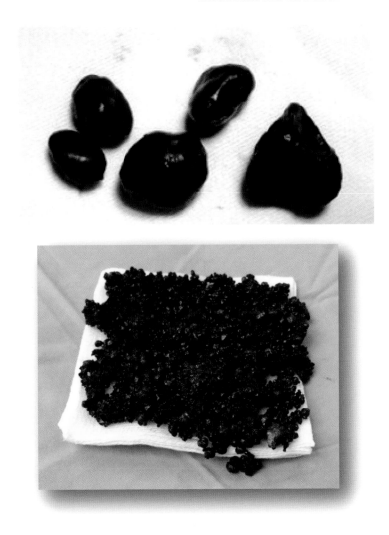

Figure 1. Pigmented gallstones.

oval-shaped, with a central dark spot (Fig. 2). Cholesterol is secreted into bile together with lecithin, where they stay in solution in the form of unilamellar vesicles or mixed micelles. As bile becomes more concentrated in the gallbladder as a result of reabsorption of electrolytes and water, bile can become supersaturated with cholesterol with the subsequent formation of cholesterol monohydrate crystals. Hence, the incidence of cholesterol gallstones is higher

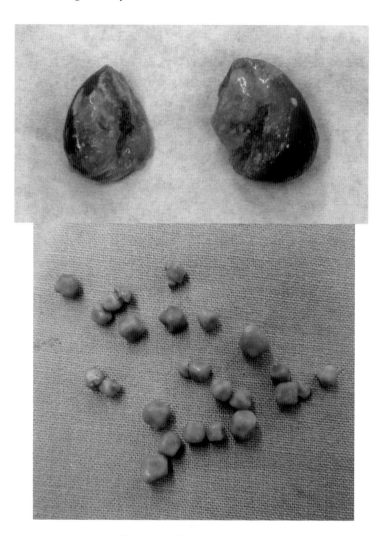

Figure 2. Cholesterol stones.

in patients who have a relatively high concentration of cholesterol in bile initially.

There are well-documented risk factors to identify those at increased risk of cholesterol gallstones:

Obesity: The metabolic syndrome of truncal obesity, insulin resistance and type II diabetes mellitus, hypertension, and hyperlipidemia is correlated closely with increased cholesterol secretion by the hepatic cells into bile, and is hence a key risk factor for the formation of cholesterol gallstones.

Pregnancy: Multiparous women have been found to have higher incidences of cholesterol gallstones, and this has been attributed to the high serum levels of progesterone during pregnancy. Progesterone's main effect on the gallbladder is to induce a state of low contractility, with resultant longer retention and concentration of bile.

Gallbladder stasis: Other causes of gallbladder stasis can also contribute to the increased risk of cholesterol gallstones formation. Patients who are on chronic total parenteral nutrition experience gallbladder stasis as a result of the lack of enteral stimulation. Increasingly, there are patients who experience rapid weight loss associated with strict caloric and fat restrictions secondary to bariatric surgery, who experience severe gallbladder stasis as well. In addition, patients who have sustained major burns or trauma, been admitted to the intensive care unit (ICU), and patients with paralysis are also at risk.

Medications: Estrogens and fibrates have been well documented to increase hepatic secretion of cholesterol, hence increasing the risk of cholesterol gallstone formation. Somatostatin analogues prejudice individuals to cholesterol gallstone formation secondary to reduced gallbladder contractility.

Hereditary: Certain genes have been found to predispose an individual to cholesterol gallstone formation, as evidenced by studies of families and twins, with at least 10 genes identified thus far.

Ileal pathology: Patients who have a diseased or resected terminal ileum experience decreased bile salt reabsorption with increased risk of gallstone formation. These include patients with Crohn's disease, prior right hemicolcetomy or small bowel resection, and other inflammatory conditions affecting the terminal ileum.

Mixed Gallstones

Mixed gallstones consist of 20–80% cholesterol by weight, and other constituents — calcium salts, bilirubin and bile pigments. These usually form as a result of enteric bacteria ascending into the gallbladder. Cholesterol stones are then colonised by the bacteria and gallbladder mucosa inflammation is

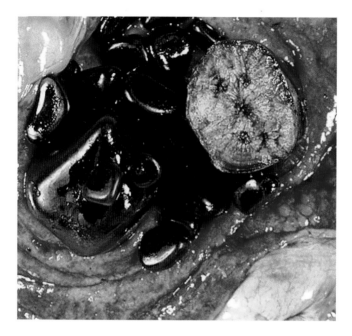

Figure 3. Mixed stones.

initiated, with the introduction of leukocytes into the reaction. Bacteria and leukocytes hydrolyse fatty acids and bilirubin conjugates, with subsequent formation of calcium salts including bilirubinate. Mixed gallstones thus usually have a cholesterol-based core, with a rim of pigmented calcium salts on the periphery (Fig. 3).

Asymptomatic Gallbladder Disease

The finding of gallstones in patients with no symptoms of biliary disease is increasingly common due to the widespread use of ultrasound for screening and computer tomography for diagnosis of vague abdominal symptoms. In the majority of asymptomatic patients, there is no indication for cholecystectomy, due to the risks of the operation outweighing potential morbidity arising from gallbladder disease in the future. The likelihood of developing symptoms or complications is approximately 1–2% per year.

There are, however, special populations who are deemed to be candidates for prophylactic cholecystectomy for asymptomatic gallstones and other gall-bladder pathologies. The following are common reasons considered to be indications:

- Sickle cell disease
- Immune system suppression
- Awaiting organ transplant
- Porcelain (calcified) gallbladder (Fig. 4)
- Gallbladder trauma
- Gallbladder polyp >10 mm in size or rapid increase in size (Fig. 5)
- Large gallstones >30 mm
- Anomalous junction of pancreatobiliary ducts
- Poorly-controlled diabetes mellitus
- Spinal cord injuries or sensory neuropathies affecting the abdomen
- Cirrhosis and portal hypertension
- Children

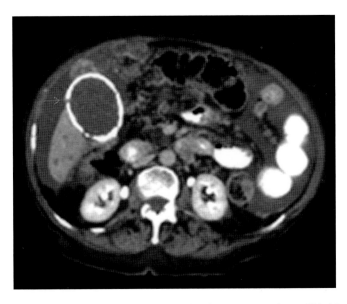

Figure 4. Axial section of a computer tomography showing a porcelain gallbladder with its calcified wall (red arrow).

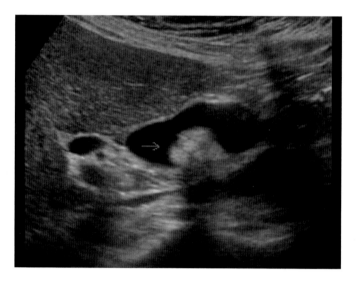

Figure 5. Large gallbladder polyp (red arrow) seen on ultrasound.

Morbid obesity may be a relative indication for prophylactic cholecystectomy especially in patients who are undergoing gastric bypass surgery, although this currently remains controversial.

This list is not exhaustive, and patients should discuss with their surgeon on their individual need for cholecystectomy based on their co-morbidities.

As gallstones are fairly common and can coexist with other intra-abdominal pathology, investigations for nonspecific and vague abdominal symptoms usually lead to their discovery. Treatment directed at these innocent bystanders are unlikely to relieve the patient's symptoms.

Symptomatic Gallstone Disease

Biliary Colic

Biliary colic is the most common indication for routine laparoscopic cholecystectomy. It is caused by the intermittent obstruction of the cystic duct by gallstone(s) (Figs. 6 and 7) with resultant gallbladder distension which in turn triggers the sensation of colicky upper abdominal pain that comes in waves.

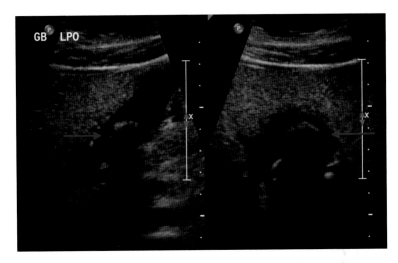

Figure 6. Ultrasound of multiple gallstones (red arrows) in a patient with biliary colic.

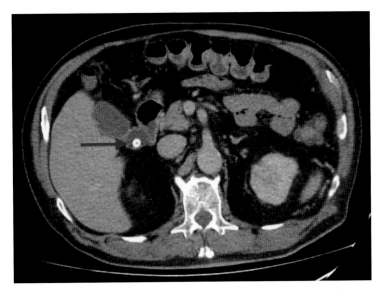

Figure 7. A solitary calcified gallstone (red arrow) in an otherwise normal gallbladder.

The pain usually resolves over 30 to 90 minutes as the obstruction is relieved and the gallbladder relaxes. Episodes of biliary colic are intermittent and erratic, and is usually localised to the epigastrium or right upper quadrant, though it may occasionally radiate to the right scapular tip. The pain is constant and is not relieved by vomiting, defecation or flatus, changes in position or anti-acid medication.

Acute Calculous Cholecystitis

This refers to inflammation of the gallbladder, and is usually precipitated by the prolonged cystic duct obstruction by gallstones (Figs. 8–11). The distension

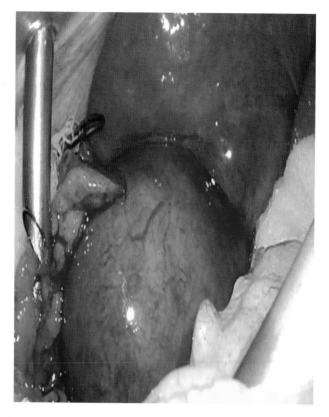

Figure 8.   Intra-operative image of acute cholecystitis. The wall is thickened, edematous and angry-looking.

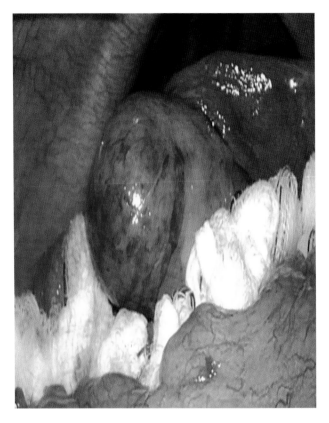

Figure 9. Another case of acute cholecystitis.

of the gallbladder causes blood flow to the gallbladder to be compromised, leading to gallbladder mucosa ischaemia and ultimately bacterial translocation, and gallbladder inflammation. In addition to the localisation of pain on the right upper quadrant, there will also be fever, localised right hypochondrium tenderness, positive Murphy's sign and biochemical evidence of inflammation and infection.

There has been controversy as to the optimal timing of laparoscopic cholecystectomy following an attack of acute cholecystitis, with some quoting a cut-off time of 72 hours from the onset of symptoms, after which dissection is theorised to be more difficult due to the inflammation. After this cut-off period, patients are treated with antibiotics and an interval

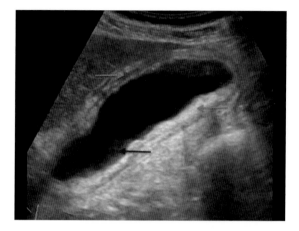

Figure 10. Ultrasound image of acute calculous cholecystitis. The red arrow indicates pericholecystic fluid. The green arrow indicates the thickened gallbladder wall. The dark blue arrow indicates a thin layer of gallstones.

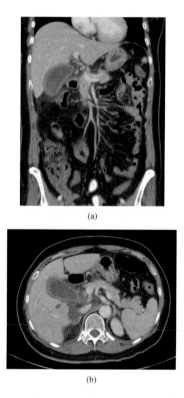

(a)

(b)

Figure 11. Computer tomographic images showing acute cholecystitis. Note the thickened gallbladder wall and pericholecystic fluid.

cholecystectomy may be planned 4 to 6 weeks later. Other surgeons though, prefer to operate on all cases of cholecystitis during the same admission regardless of time from presentation. The authors follow the latter approach, which we feel decreases total hospitalisation costs and prevents the recurrence of cholecystitis during the interval between the first attack and the elective operation.

Complicated Gallstone Disease

Gallbladder Empyema and Gangrenous Cholecystitis

Empyema of the gallbladder and gangrenous cholecystitis are conditions that represent an escalation of disease in patients with cholecystitis.

Empyema occurs when the gallbladder becomes filled with pus due to severe bacterial infection (Fig. 12). The symptoms and signs are usually more severe than that of acute cholecystitis. A globular mass may be appreciated on palpation of the right hypochondrium, which represents a tense, enlarged gallbladder that may be encased with adherent omentum.

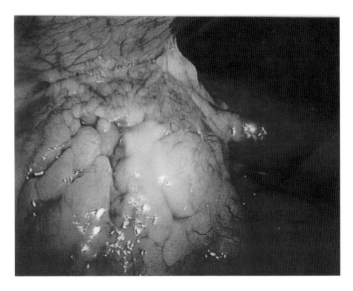

Figure 12.   Gallbladder empyema with a severe inflammatory reaction involving omentum. This patient had a palpable mass in the right hypochondrium on clinical examination.

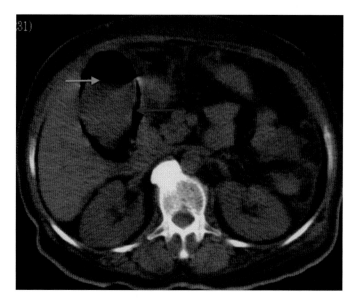

Figure 13.   Axial section of a computer tomography image showing gangrenous cholecystitis. The green arrow indicates the air-fluid level, and the red arrow indicates air within the gallbladder wall, or emphysematous gallbladder wall.

Gangrenous cholecystitis refers to gallbladder wall necrosis secondary to ischaemia, which in itself can lead to gallbladder perforation and resultant pericholecystic abscess formation or bilious peritonitis. Gangrenous cholecystitis is usually a radiological diagnosis, as evidenced by non-enhancing mucosa on contrast computer tomography scan, or thinning of the gallbladder wall seen on ultrasound or computer tomography (Fig. 13). Intra-operatively, it can be recognised as patches of gangrene on an acutely inflamed gallbladder (Fig. 14). Once gallbladder perforation occurs, the patient may actually have a transient relief of his/her abdominal pain as the gallbladder discharges its contents into the peritoneal cavity. However, the patient's clinical course can quickly deteriorate as peritonitis sets in. Development of generalised abdominal rebound tenderness and guarding, with increasing haemodynamic instability can give clues to the diagnosis.

In both these conditions, one can expect a more severe haematological and biochemical inflammatory response. Both these conditions require urgent surgical treatment; alternatively, a percutaneous cholecystotomy can be performed as a temporising measure for patients too ill to undergo surgery.

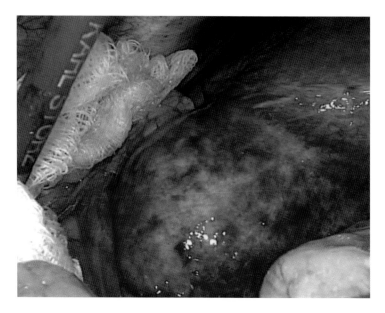

Figure 14.   Intra-operative empyema. Note the thickened and ischaemic gallbladder wall.

Chronic Cholecystitis

Over the long term, repeated attacks of acute cholecystitis and localised ischaemia caused by gallstones pressing upon the gallbladder wall can lead to chronic cholecystitis. In this condition, the gallbladder undergoes fibrosis, shrinks, and loses its contractile function. The contracted gallbladder may become adhered to adjacent organs as the disease progresses.

The diagnosis can be suspected by a submitted history of repeated episodes of acute cholecystitis that were treated conservatively, or a pattern of severe biliary colic. Radiologically, the gallbladder can be seen as thick-walled and shrunken (Fig. 15).

Choledocholithiasis and Cholangitis

Choledocholithiasis refers to the presence of gallstones in the common bile duct, the majority of which originate from the gallbladder, with or without obstruction of bile flow. The spiral valves of the cystic duct normally retain gallstones within the gallbladder, but become obliterated with repeated bouts of gallstone impaction at the cystic duct, allowing the passage of gallstones

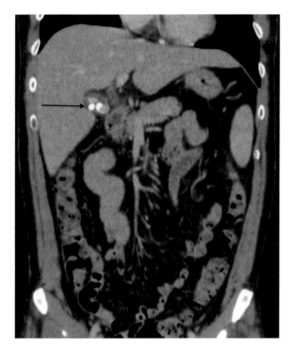

Figure 15.   The gallbladder (black arrow) is filled radio-opaque gallstones and is fibrotic and shrunken as a result of chronic inflammation.

into the common bile duct. Stones in the common bile duct may be asymptomatic if small enough, but may also impact at the distal common bile duct where it narrows, causing biliary colic similar to that caused by cystic duct obstruction (Fig. 16). Scleral icterus, and biochemical evidence of jaundice and deranged hepatic enzymes can result from the backpressure of bile secondary to the obstruction.

Cholangitis is the purulent inflammation of the biliary tree, caused as a result of bacterial overgrowth in stagnant bile precipitated by the presence of biliary obstruction and stasis. More uncommonly, cholangitis can result from strictures caused by inflammatory conditions or malignancy. In addition to the symptoms and signs of biliary obstruction, patients with cholangitis will also have fever, haematological and biochemical evidence of bacterial infection. If left untreated, patients may progress rapidly to septic shock.

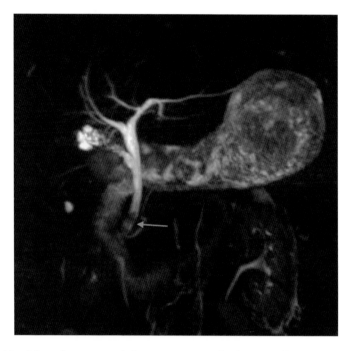

Figure 16. Magnetic resonance cholangiopancreatography showing gallstones and distal common bile duct stone (green arrow), that are causing proximal bile duct obstruction and dilation.

Preoperative or postoperative endoscopic retrograde cholangiopancreatography (ERCP) with sphincterotomy are options, as is a single laparoscopic operation, to remove the gallbladder and explore the common bile duct (Fig. 17). The decision for treatment depends strongly on the availability of local expertise.

We prefer a pre-operative ERCP to clear the biliary stones, failing which biliary stent placement is performed to relieve the obstruction (Fig. 18). This is followed by a same-admission laparoscopic cholecystectomy approach, usually within 24–48 hours. This allows the patient to be treated within the same admission, and the sedation from the ERCP procedure usually allows the patient to transit into anaesthesia for surgery seamlessly. While ERCP is not without its own set of complications, we find that in our hands it is more straightforward, and a much less morbid option than laparoscopic common bile duct exploration.

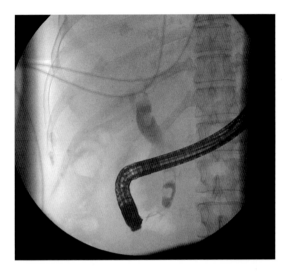

Figure 17. ERCP showing multiple stones in the common bile duct.

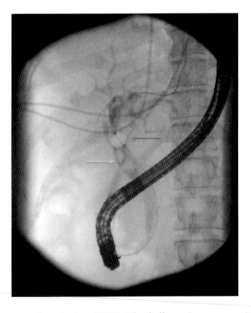

Figure 18. Stone extraction during ERCP. The balloon (green arrow) has been inflated proximal to the common bile duct stones (yellow arrow), in preparation of balloon extraction. The balloon will be pulled distally; with the aim of trawling the stones pass the sphincter of Oddi into the duodenum. Balloon extraction is usually preceded by sphincterotomy to allow passage of the common bile duct stones.

In the event of a complicated ERCP or haemodynamic instability precluding sedation needed for ERCP, the more pressing issue of biliary drainage can be achieved with percutaneous drainage of the biliary system to allow for patient stabilisation. ERCP can be re-attempted once the patient is stabilised before laparoscopic cholecystectomy is performed. Otherwise, the laparoscopic common bile duct exploration can be performed in the same setting as laparoscopic cholecystectomy.

Multiple or impacted common bile duct stones may necessitate repeat ERCP attempts for stenting and stone extraction (Fig. 19). These multiple ERCP attempts may be spaced by intervals of a few weeks, to allow for resolution of inflammation and dissolution of the biliary stones. An in-depth discussion on ERCPs and biliary stone management is beyond the scope of this book.

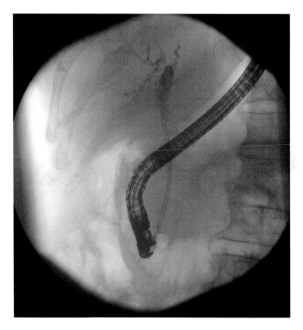

Figure 19. Stent placement in the common bile duct after failed stone extraction. The proximal end of the stent is placed above the obstruction, and the distal tip rests within the duodenum, allowing biliary flow despite the presence of remnant common bile duct stones.

Gallstone Pancreatitis

Gallstones are the leading cause of pancreatitis, and the diagnosis of gallstone-induced pancreatitis warrants the removal of the gallbladder. A gallstone that becomes impacted at the ampulla of Vater may temporarily obstruct the pancreatic duct, leading to activation of pancreatic proteases, with ensuing auto-digestion and pancreatitis (Fig. 20). The pain associated with pancreatitis is distinctly different from that of biliary pain, and is described as sharp, severe, continuous, and located in the epigastrium with radiation to the back.

Pancreatitis can be mild, moderate or severe, based on the patient's clinical course and development of local or systemic complications, and the presence of end-organ dysfunction. In mild to moderate case of pancreatitis, the surgery can be performed within the same admission. However, in more severe cases, it is prudent to await the recovery of the patient from his/her pancreatitis before planning for surgery.

Mirizzi's Syndrome

This refers to a special situation where a gallstone lodged in the cystic duct or Hartmann's pouch causes compression of the common hepatic duct to

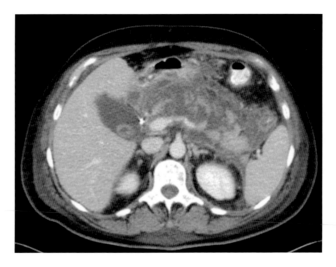

Figure 20. Pancreatitis with necrosis of the head and body, with a gallstone in the gallbladder. The likely aetiology here would be gallstone-induced pancreatitis.

varying degrees. Pre-operative ERCP with stenting can be attempted; otherwise careful laparoscopic dissection by an experienced surgeon can attempt the removal of gallbladder. The degree of severity of Mirizzi's syndrome can range from simple compression, to fistulisation into the common hepatic duct, and determines the optimal surgical approach taken.

Special Populations

Children

In children with haematological conditions such as thalassemia and sickle cell anaemia, a high turnover of red abnormal red blood cells results in additional bile pigments produced — which then predisposes them to the early development of pigmented gallstones. Laparoscopic cholecystectomy has been shown to be a safe option with similar results as compared to adults.

Cirrhosis

Patients with Child-Pugh-Turcotte Class A or B cirrhosis and symptomatic gallstone disease are considered candidates for laparoscopic cholecystectomy. In patients with Class C cirrhosis, medical management is preferred especially if the patient is a transplant candidate. These patients are at a much higher risk of anaesthetic and surgical complications, and the gallbladder will be removed together with the diseased liver during the transplant procedure. Due to their more severe disease state, Class C cirrhotic patients are at a higher priority and can expect a relatively shorter waiting time.

Pregnancy

Pregnant patients are generally treated with medical therapy before attempting laparoscopic cholecystectomy as a last resort for patients who fail medical therapy.

The second trimester is considered the safest period to undergo surgery, but should be carried out by experienced surgeons in high volume centres. Special positioning and anaesthetic considerations also have to be factored in for this special group of patients.

Absolute Contraindications

Inability to Tolerate General Anaesthesia, Pneumopritoneum

Patients who are too ill to undergo general anaesthesia are unable to have gallbladder surgery performed on them. These patients usually have severe cardiac or respiratory conditions that preclude general anaesthesia, or are haemodynamically unstable from an acute medical condition.

In patients whose medical conditions prevent them from tolerating the pneumoperitoneum needed for laparoscopic cholecystectomy, the traditional open cholecystectomy is the preferred option.

Uncontrolled Coagulopathy

Patients who are coagulopathic need to have their clotting profile normalised or controlled before surgery can be attempted. A coagulopathic state may arise either as a result of medical anti-coagulation, or secondary to disease states like disseminated intravascular coagulation in patients with sepsis. These usually require the use of blood products, vitamin K supplementation, or simply suspension of the offending drug, depending on the exact aetiology of coagulopathy and urgency of operative intervention.

Patients who are on anti-platelet therapy for their cardiac or neurovascular condition may need to suspend their medication for a few days prior to surgery if an elective procedure is planned. If emergent intervention is required, the surgeons will then have to take necessary steps intraoperatively to mitigate the risk of bleeding.

Gallbladder Cancer

The pre-operative diagnosis of gallbladder cancer is an absolute contraindication to laparoscopic cholecystectomy, due to the risk of tumour spillage and inadequate resection margins. If cancer is diagnosed intra-operatively, then the procedure should be converted to the open approach.

Gallbladder cancer is usually locally advanced or metastatic if diagnosed pre-operatively by radiological studies (Fig. 21). Either a radical cholecystectomy (including resection of segments 4 and 5, and hepatoduodenal lymphadenectomy) or a palliative bypass procedure is performed, depending on the possibility of cure.

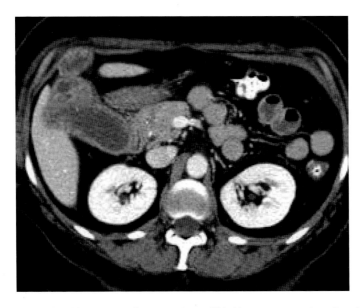

Figure 21. Gallbladder cancer: a heterogeneous gallbladder mass is seen invading the adjacent liver parenchyma.

Gallbladder cancer is not uncommonly diagnosed post-operatively on histological examination after laparoscopic cholecystectomy has been performed for a presumed benign condition, such as gallstones or polyp(s). The crucial point is whether the cancer has invaded the submucosa; current evidence suggests that cancers invading the submucosa will require a radical cholecystectomy to reduce local recurrence and disease progression, while tumours not involving the submucosa can be treated satisfactorily with simple laparoscopic cholecystectomy. The presence of tumor at the resected cystic duct margin and lymphatic invasion also indicate the need for further radical resection if possible. The staging, surgical options, and adjuvant therapy for gallbladder cancer are beyond the scope of this book.

Diagnosis

Gallstones can give rise to a spectrum of pathological processes that cause patients to present with symptoms. In addition, gallstone disease is at times difficult to differentiate from diseases involving other organs in the vicinity, which further complicates matters.

Symptoms and Signs of Gallstone Pathology

Symptoms can initially be vague, such as upper abdominal discomfort and bloating and flatulence after meals. These usually reflect uncomplicated gallstone disease in which intermittent obstruction of the cystic duct by the gallstone(s) result in the occurrence of symptoms, otherwise known as biliary colic (Fig. 1). Patients usually have a normal physical examination at this point in the disease spectrum.

As the disease progresses to inflammation of the gallbladder, or acute cholecystitis, symptoms become more severe and results in right upper abdominal pain, which may be worse on inspiration. Vomiting and rigors may also be a feature at this point. Patients will have fever and tenderness over the right hypochondrium. The gallbladder may become palpable if suitably engorged with mucus (mucocele) or pus (empyema), although most chronically inflamed gallbladders are contracted and non-palpable. Murphy's sign, which refers to a patient catching his/her breath during inspiration when the right hypochondrium is palpated, is characteristic for cholecystitis.

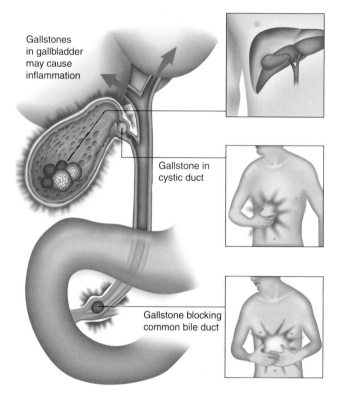

Gallstones in gallbladder may cause inflammation

Gallstone in cystic duct

Gallstone blocking common bile duct

Figure 1. Presence of gallstones in different portions of the biliary tree can produce symptoms of colicky pain, nausea, and flatulence.

In the event of choledocholithiasis, patients may experience jaundice, or yellowing of the mucous membranes (Fig. 2). This is most easily appreciated by examining the sclera and oral cavity. Tea-coloured urine is also a common sign. If complicated by cholangitis, the abdominal pain, chills, rigors and fever may become more prominent. The classic Charcot's triad of cholangitis consists of fever, right hypochondrium pain and jaundice. As sepsis progresses, patients may start to exhibit haemodynamic instability, with increased heart rate and lowered blood pressure. Acute mental status changes such as lethargy, confusion and altered level of consciousness are seen in severe cases. This completes the Reynold's pentad of cholangitis.

Gallstone-induced pancreatitis results in a central, deep-seated sharp pain that may radiate towards the back. Extreme epigastric tenderness may also be a feature. Mild cases are usually haemodynamically stable, but patients with

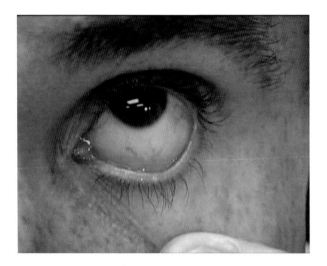

Figure 2. Scleral jaundice secondary to choledocholithiasis.

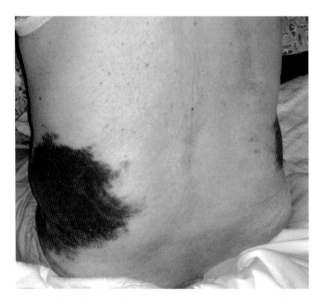

Figure 3. Grey-Turner's sign, flank ecchymosis from retroperitoneal haemorrhage.

severe pancreatitis can present in shock. In addition, severe pancreatitis can cause retroperitoneal haemorrhage with flank ecchymosis (Grey-Turner's sign) or periumbilical ecchymosis (Cullen's sign) (Figs. 3 and 4).

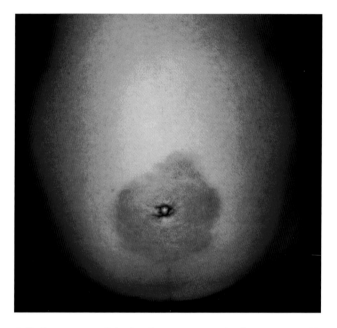

Figure 4. Cullen's sign, periumbilical ecchymosis as a result of retroperitoneal haemorrhage.

Biochemical Investigations

In patients with suspected complications from gallstones, blood tests should routinely include a full blood count with differential count, liver function panel, renal function panel, amylase and lipase.

Blood tests during biliary colic are usually completely normal. Patients with cholesterol stones frequently have concomitant fatty liver, which may cause a mild rise in the liver enzymes alanine transaminase (ALT) and aspartate transaminase (AST).

During an episode of acute cholecystitis, inflammatory markers are usually raised; these include white blood cells with neutrophilia and a left shift, C-reactive protein (CRP), prolactin and erythrocyte sedimentation rate (ESR). Liver enzymes are usually normal at this point, though severe gallbladder inflammation may cause a transient rise in the transaminases secondary to sepsis.

In the presence of significant biliary obstruction from choledocholelithiasis, an acute rise in the serum level of ALT and AST is observed. Within a few hours, total serum bilirubin will be increased, with the direct component being disproportionately raised. As the obstruction persists, alkaline phosphatase (ALP) and gamma-glutamyl-transferase (GGT) are liver enzymes that become commonly raised as well. With chronic common bile duct obstruction, the prothrombin time (PT) will be raised, secondary to a depletion of vitamin K, the absorption of which is bile-dependent. In the presence of cholangitis, raised inflammatory markers in combination to markers of biliary obstruction are typically present.

Acute pancreatitis by any aetiology will cause a rise in serum amylase and lipase. Serum lipase stays elevated for a longer period of time, and may be more sensitive for diagnosis of pancreatitis when there is a delay in patient presentation. Chronic pancreatitis may not have any elevation in serum amylase or lipase levels, due to the "burning-out"of the pancreas. However, gallstones do not classically cause chronic pancreatitis; alcohol abuse, drugs and autoimmune pancreatitis are far more common causes.

In severe cases of cholangitis or pancreatitis, shock may ensue with anaerobic metabolism resulting in raised serum lactate levels and metabolic acidosis. There are scoring systems (such as Ranson's, APACHE II etc.) that serve to assess the severity of pancreatitis by measuring multi-organ dysfunction. Pre-renal failure is also seen in shock and manifests as raised serum urea and creatinine levels, with the urea: creatinine ratio more than 20. These scores serve as a clinical guide but should not replace a proper history, physical examination and assessment of each individual patient when making a clinical judgment.

Serial testing over days is useful in evaluating the clinical course of patients and the need for emergent intervention. Decreasing serum levels of bilirubin and hepatic enzymes may reflect spontaneous passage of an obstructing stone. Contrariwise, increasing serum levels of bilirubin, hepatic enzymes and leukocytosis despite antibiotic therapy may indicate refractory ascending cholangitis with need for urgent intervention.

Radiological and Endoscopic Investigations

To make the diagnosis of gallstone disease, a full history and physical examination is key. Armed with initial differential diagnoses, specialised tests can then be ordered to either confirm or exclude diagnoses.

Abdominal Radiography

Upright and supine abdominal radiographs may be occasionally helpful in suggesting a diagnosis of gallstone disease.

Black pigment or mixed gallstones might comprise of adequate calcium to appear radiopaque on plain radiography. Air within the biliary tree may imply the presence of a biliary-enteric fistula or ascending cholangitis with gas-forming organisms. Calcification of the gallbladder wall (porcelain gallbladder) is indicative of severe chronic cholecystitis, and alerts the surgeon to the possibility of carcinoma development.

However, where healthcare facilities are satisfactory, abdominal radiography's main role in evaluating patients with suspected gallstone disease is to exclude other causes of acute abdominal pain. These include conditions such chronic calcific pancreatitis, intestinal obstruction, visceral perforation or renal stones.

Transabdominal Ultrasound

The most commonly used and effective method of diagnosing gallstone disease is a transabdominal ultrasound. It has the advantage of being cheap, non-invasive, portable, and provides a commendable level of sensitivity and specificity. It also does not expose patients to radiation (hence safe in pregnancy) and intravenous contrast.

Its disadvantages include being operator-dependent and relative lack of availability after-hours. Thick abdominal walls in obese patients also reduce the quality of images available to the radiographer. Whilst gallstones greater than 2 mm are easily detected, biliary sludge or microlithiasis tend to be more obscure. Furthermore, anatomy of the distal common bile duct and pancreas can be obscured by bowel gas, reducing its level of accuracy.

Gallstones appear as echogenic foci in the gallbladder wall, move freely with positional changes and cast an acoustic shadow (Fig. 5).

Uncomplicated acute cholecystitis can be easily diagnosed with ultrasonography. The sonographic features of acute cholecystitis include pericholecystic fluid, gallbladder distention (>5 cm), gallbladder wall thickening (>5 mm) and a positive sonographic Murphy's sign (Fig. 6). Ultrasound can also reliably exclude other hepatic parenchymal pathology that may be causing the patient's symptoms, such as hepatic abscesses or tumours.

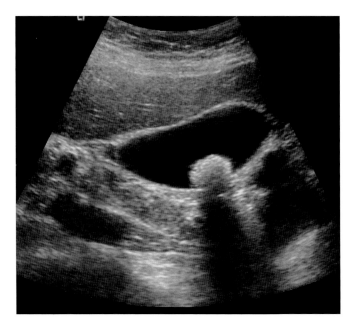

Figure 5. Ultrasound of uncomplicated cholelithiasis. The gallbladder wall is thin and is not inflamed, and there is no pericholecystic fluid. There is a single large calculus with posterior acoustic shadowing.

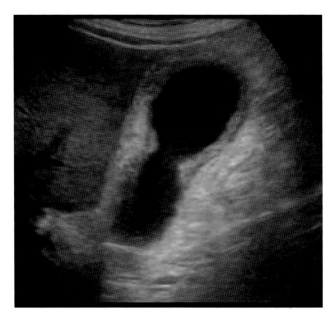

Figure 6. Acute cholecystitis. Note the thickened gallbladder wall and sludge along the wall.

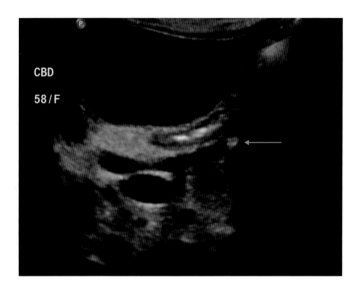

Figure 7. A common bile duct stone (green arrow) in a patient who presented with jaundice and abdominal pain.

The sensitivity of ultrasonography for common bile duct (CBD) stones is far from ideal. These are due to a few factors: (1) duodenal gas conceals the distal portion of the CBD, where most impacted CBD stones are located; (2) the curvature of the CBD may induce refraction and reflection of the ultrasound wave; and (3) the depth of the distal CBD could be past the optimal focal point of the transducer (Fig. 7). CBD dilation identified on ultrasound is an indirect indicator of CBD obstruction, but may be absent if the obstruction was of recent onset. Furthermore, in elderly patients whose bile ducts dilate as a result of normal ageing, the accuracy of CBD dilation in diagnosing CBD stones is hampered.

Endoscopic Ultrasound

Endoscopic ultrasound (EUS) involves using an ultrasound probe mounted on an endoscope to achieve ultrasonic images of better quality and resolution compared to transabdominal ultrasound (Fig. 8). However, it is an invasive procedure and has a complication rate comparable to diagnostic gastroscopy. It is highly operator-dependent and requires intensive training to be proficient, limiting its availability to a few specialised centres. It is not

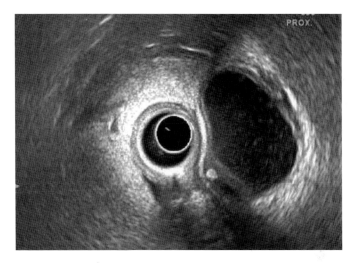

Figure 8. EUS demonstrating a small stone in the gallbladder.

usually performed for the majority of disease involving the gallbladder; its use is more relevant when the cause of biliary dilation is occult, and for accurate nodal and local staging of pancreatic and gastric cancer. However, it can on occasion detect common bile duct sludge and irregularities not observed with other modalities. In addition, it can be used to guide diagnostic fine-needle aspiration cytology or therapeutic treatments of pancreatic pseudocysts and abscesses.

Laparoscopic Ultrasound

Laparoscopic ultrasound is a technique that has been recently applied in some centres to evaluate the bile duct during laparoscopic cholecystectomy for cholelithiasis. Patients who are deemed to be at high or intermediate risk of choledocholithiasis may be suitable, and this technique might become routine in evaluating the CBD in lieu of intraoperative cholangiogram.

Computer Tomography

Though not the initial choice in biliary colic, computer-tomography (CT) scans are increasingly being used to diagnose gallstone disease as it offers a few key advantages. It is not operator-dependent, relatively quick and available even after-hours in most institutions, and can provide a good amount of anatomical characterisation, including the demonstration of distal CBD stones. It may also be able to confirm or exclude other abdominal pathologies, and help further characterise complications of gallstone disease. Its disadvantages include the relative higher cost, radiation and risk of allergy due to the use of contrast material. Patients with a decreased baseline kidney function are also at increased risk of suffering transient or permanent kidney damage from the contrast material. CT scans may also miss small gallstones, although CT scanners boasting higher resolution and thinner cuts are gradually solving this problem.

On CT, gallstones appear as single or multiple filling defects within the gallbladder. Depending on their composition and etiology, gallstones can either be densely calcified, rim calcified, laminated, having a central nidus of calcification, or as soft-tissue density (Figs. 9 and 10). The features of acute cholecystitis are similar to ultrasonography. Radiolucent stones that have the same density as bile cannot be visualised, and some small non-calcified stones may be confused with polyps.

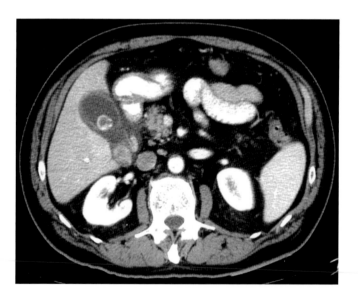

Figure 9. A computer tomography scan showing cholecystitis: gallstones, thickened gallbladder wall, pericholecystic fluid, pericholecystic fat stranding.

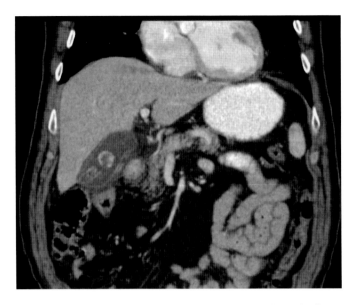

Figure 10. Computer tomography scan of a different patient with similar features of acute cholecystitis.

Magnetic Resonance Imaging

Magnetic resonance imaging (MRI), or magnetic resonance cholangiopancreatography (MRCP) scans have found increased use in complex cases, where US and CT scans fail to provide a definite diagnosis but disease involving the biliary tree is still strongly suspected (Figs. 11 and 12). In other cases, it can be used to further delineate anatomy in patients in whom surgery is being considered. Its advantages are increased resolution, characterisation of anatomy and lack of radiation.

However, it is expensive, relatively slow, and its availability may be an issue in some centres. Unstable patients are also not candidates for a MRI scan due to the prolonged period when the physician loses direct contact with the patient during the scan. The contrast material used in MRI scans may also cause scarring of tissue in patients with decreased kidney function. Some stones may be indistinguishable from polyps, and smaller stones may be missed due to respiratory or motion artifacts.

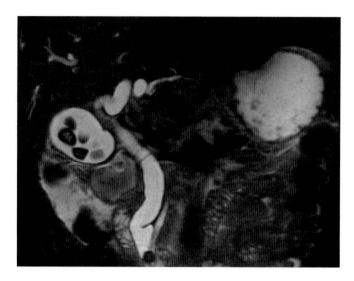

Figure 11. Cholelithiasis and choledocholithiasis with biliary dilation demonstrated by MRCP.

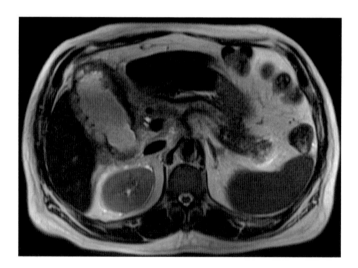

Figure 12.   MRCP showing abnormal thickening of the gallbladder wall, suggestive of severe infection.

Endoscopic Retrograde Cholangiopancreatography

Endoscopic retrograde cholangiopancreatography (ERCP) is an invasive procedure in which a side-viewing endoscope is inserted via the patient's mouth to visualise the biliary tree. It has both diagnostic and therapeutic applications, although its use has been increasingly limited to therapeutic purposes, given the diagnostic efficacy of MRCP. By cannulating the ampulla of Vater and injecting contrast material, the endoscopist is able to visualise the external and internal biliary tree and pancreatic duct anatomy. Stones appear as filling defects in the opacified ducts (Fig. 13). Applications include removal of common bile duct stones, dilatation and stenting of strictures, and sphincterotomies (Figs. 14–16). It has notable complications, such as pancreatitis, bleeding, perforation and failure of therapy.

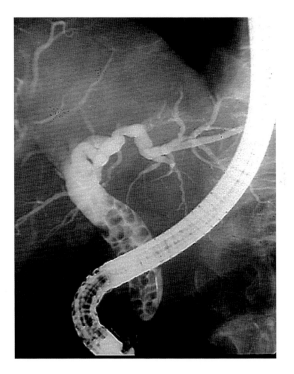

Figure 13. ERCP showing multiple small gallstones within the common bile duct causing upstream obstruction and dilation.

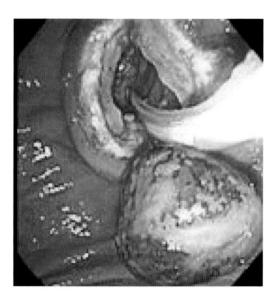

Figure 14.   Extraction of a mixed stone following a large sphincterotomy.

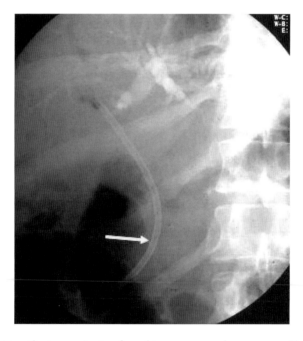

Figure 15.   Plastic stent *in situ* after sphincterotomy and stone removal by ERCP.

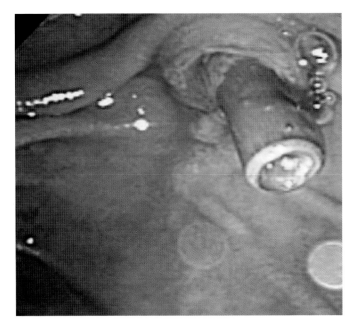

Figure 16. Endoscopic view of a plastic stent placed in the common bile duct, with its tip within the duodenal lumen. This allows for drainage of bile to bypass obstructions secondary to gallstones, strictures, or tumours.

Scintigraphy

A rarely performed investigation locally is the cholescintigraphy scan, a nuclear imaging procedure to evaluate the health and function of the gallbladder. It is also known as a hepatoiminodiacetic acid (HIDA), paraisopropyl iminodiacetic acid (PIPIDA), or diisopropyl iminodiacetic acid (DISIDA) scan, depending on the nuclear agent used. The radioactive tracer is injected intravenously, and given time to circulate and be processed by the liver, where it will be excreted into the biliary system. Failure of gallbladder visualisation is highly suggestive that the patient has cholecystitis or cystic duct obstruction secondary to a gallstone, hence preventing the filling up of the gallbladder with the radioactive tracer. Gallbladder ejection fraction can also be measured, which may be decreased in cholelithiasis or chronic cholecystitis.

This test is usually done after an ultrasound of the abdomen fails to detect the presence of any gallstones or abnormalities, in an attempt to establish a cause of right upper quadrant pain. This test is not generally performed as a first-line investigation due to its cost and invasiveness. In addition, it provides little information about non-obstructing cholelithiasis and other pathological states.

Pre-operative Assessment

Careful pre-operative planning allows for any potential problems or contraindications to surgery to be resolved before the operation. It decreases the rate of cancelled surgeries, and improves patients' confidence and satisfaction with the peri-operative experience.

Risk Assessment

Laparoscopic cholecystectomy is considered a moderate-risk procedure. Patients under the age of 40 with no significant medical history can usually be cleared for surgery with nothing more than a questionnaire. Patients with noteworthy comorbidities however, require pre-operative testing of relevant physiological systems to investigate potential contraindications to surgery. It also allows remedial measures to be undertaken to reduce the potential complications as a result of surgery. Age is a marker for decreased physiological reserve, and for the increasing incidence of comorbidities in patients.

Cardiovascular issues are probably the most common pre-operative concern encountered and also the most lethal. Patients with a history of angina, myocardial infarction, heart failure, cerebrovascular accident or peripheral vascular disease have a significant risk of peri-operative heart attack and/or stroke. Furthermore, many of these patients are on anti-platelets and anti-coagulants, which may need to be stopped or bridged, hence complicating the peri-operative preparation.

Patients with pulmonary disease such as chronic obstructive pulmonary disease may find themselves at higher risk of post-operative pneumonia or extubation failure, requiring prolonged periods in the intensive care unit. The splinting of the diaphragm from the pneumoperitoneum created intra-operatively lends itself to higher airway pressures needed to ventilate the patient, with a resultant increased risk of pneumothorax.

Renal dysfunction and failure is increasingly prevalent, thanks to the incidence of diabetes and longer survival periods of renal failure patients due to renal replacement therapies. Patients with renal failure usually have concomitant cardiovascular issues. Scheduling of surgery is hindered by the need to factor in the patient's dialysis requirements, and there is increased risk of fluid overload and electrolyte imbalances. In addition, platelet dysfunction secondary to uraemia escalates the jeopardy of intra-operative and post-operative bleeding.

Patients with congenital or acquired disorders of bleeding and coagulation may need peri-operative intervention, or have the operation postponed if the deficiency cannot be rectified in time. Patients with platelet or coagulation factor(s) deficiency or dysfunction may require peri-operative transfusions of blood product(s). Conversely, patients with increased risk of thrombosis due to inherited defects or acquired conditions usually require intra-operative mechanical prophylaxis with intermittent pneumatic calf-pumps, and early post-operative anticoagulation.

Obese patients are well recognised to have increased risk of cardiovascular, respiratory, thrombotic, and wound complications during and after surgery. Diabetic patients similarly face an increase risk of cardiovascular and wound complications. Pre-operative weight-loss regimes, and glycaemic control can help mitigate, but not eliminate these risks.

Having patients attend a pre-operative anaesthetic assessment clinic increases the chances that impending issues will be picked up after a systemic review. The relevant specialists should be consulted if there is any doubt at all on the part of the surgeon or the anaesthetist as to the optimal peri-operative management plan.

Pre-operative Education

The main aim is for the patient to be fully aware of his/her condition, so as to empower them to make an informed decision. Surgeons cannot force a particular treatment onto a patient, although they do have enormous sway in helping patients decide on whether to proceed with treatment. When patients feel knowledgeable and in control, they ultimately are more satisfied with the entire peri-operative experience.

Patients should have their condition explained to them in simple layman terms to avoid alienating them with medical jargon. Next, treatment options with the pros and cons of each option should be explained in turn, specific to the patient and his/her particular condition and comorbidities; this would include the potential consequences of refusing treatment, and alternative options available. All potential complications including the possibility of conversion to an open procedure and mortality should be carefully discussed as well. The likely site of incisions, duration of post-operative pain, and expected time before discharge and subsequent return to normal activities can be discussed to better help patients manage their expectations.

It is important for surgeons to clear up any questions and doubts that patients may have prior to their surgery. Further effort must similarly be taken to address patients' concerns post-operatively.

It is routine for patients to fast for at least 8 hours prior to their elective surgery. Some classes of anti-hypertensive medications will have to be omitted on the morning of surgery, while others should be continued. Diabetic medications are usually discontinued on the morning of surgery to prevent hypoglycaemia. Anti-platelets and anti-coagulants, if deemed necessary to be omitted, should cease a few days to a week prior to surgery, depending on the specific drug in question. The decision to continue or omit medications is individually ascertained and should be advised by the anaesthetist in discussion with the surgeon.

To decrease the risk of wound infections, patients should be discouraged from shaving the incision sites. Also, body washing with chlorhexidine or soaps may help decrease the incidence of wound infections. Proper explanation for the rationale of these pre-operative steps helps to improve compliance.

Operative Procedure

Before the first incision is made, adequate preparation is necessary to ensure a smooth operation. This process is usually protocoled, and ensures that the correct operation is being performed on the correct patient. In addition, the surgeon must check that all necessary equipment is set up and available before initiating the operation. Rushing to begin the operation without ensuring proper set-up compromises the safety of the patient, and usually leads to unnecessary angst and stress for the surgical team.

Positioning of Patient

Patients are placed in a supine position, usually with the right arm tucked in and flushed against their torso. Their left arm can be tucked in also, but is usually positioned at right angles to the torso on an arm-board to provide easier intravenous access for the anaesthetist. The right arm is tucked in specifically to provide for standing space for the assistant in the event of a conversion to open surgery. This allows for the surgeon to operate from the right side of the patient, with additional space to the surgeon's left for an assistant to perform retraction of the right costal margin.

Warming mats placed beneath the patient are routinely used in most institutions to mitigate heat loss from the patient during the operation. Warmed air insufflators to create a cushion of warm air between the sheets and the patient's lower limbs are used for the same effect.

The supine position is the most benign due to the relative lack of created pressure points that may increase the risk of pressure sores. The relative short duration of a laparoscopic cholecystectomy also safeguards against the development of any iatrogenic pressure sores intra-operatively.

Cleansing and Draping

As per all abdominal operations, patients are cleaned from nipple level to mid-thigh. We prefer chlorhexidine-alcohol preparations, though iodine-based preparations have the advantage of delineating clearly the areas that have been cleansed. In particular, the right side of the abdomen should be cleansed laterally to the junction of the patient's body and the bed. This includes the abdominal wall involved in a Kocher's incision in the sterile field, so additional cleansing is not required in the event of conversion to an open procedure.

The cleanliness of the umbilicus for any laparoscopic procedure cannot be over-emphasised. Due to personal hygiene practices (or the lack thereof) and/or body habitus, the umbilicus is a common repository of debris consisting of sloughed keratin, clothing fabric and microorganisms. Cotton-tipped sticks dipped in chlorhexidine are commonly used in clearing deep-seated debris, and alcohol swabs can be used for flatter navels. Failure to pay proper attention to the sterility of this area significantly increases the risk of surgical site infection at the peri-umbilical incision.

Drapes should expose just the top of the costal margin and the xiphoid process, whilst extending to the right laterally to the mid-axillary line. This facilitates the placement of the lateral most laparoscopic port. It also allows for a lateral Kocher's (subcostal) incision that may be required in complex converted cases. The inferior edge of the drapes should be at least 2 cm below the umbilicus, which allows for enough space even if a sub-umbilical incision is made for the insertion of the laparoscope.

Positioning of Surgeon, Assistants and Camera System

High-definition television systems have become the norm in most laparoscopic procedures, with a number of manufacturers providing comparable products. An in-depth account of camera system workings is detailed in the Appendix.

The television monitor is positioned to the side of the patient's right shoulder, tilted towards his/her right hypochondrium. This allows for a straight line between the surgeon, area of interest (right hypochondrium) and the monitor, for improved ergonomics.

The surgeon stands on the left side of the patient, just below the level of the umbilicus, with his body tilted towards the patient's right hypochondrium and facing the video monitor. From this spot, he is well positioned to control both working ports.

The camera assistant stands just behind the left shoulder of the surgeon, often having to manipulate the laparoscope from a slightly awkward position so as to stay clear of the surgeon's left arm. The camera assistant usually holds the camera head base with his/her right hand from below, with his/her left hand toggling the fibre-optic cable to manoeuvre the viewing perspective, and to capture images by operating the controls on the camera head. In the case of a coaxial camera head system, both hands are also needed to control the up-down and left-right dials on the camera head (Fig. 1).

Fogging of the laparoscope lens is a common source of hindrance for the surgical team. It is primarily caused by the condensation of warmer

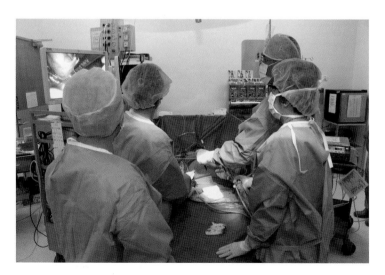

Figure 1. Positioning during surgery. The patient is lying supine with the head further from the foreground. (A) is the surgeon, standing on the left side of the patient facing the patient's right shoulder. (B) is the camera assistant. (C) is the first assistant providing cephalic retraction of the gallbladder. (D) is the scrub nurse.

water molecules present in the peritoneal cavity onto the colder surface of the lens. This can be somewhat mitigated by pre-heating the laparoscope in a special heating unit that is part of most camera systems. We find the use of a sterile thermo-flask filled with near boiling water for intermittent warming of the laparoscope during the operation very effective. A piece of gauze is placed at the bottom of the flask to prevent scratch injury to the delicate laparoscope lens.

Anti-fogging solutions that are applied to the lens by way of a sponge are also readily available, but not as successful in our experience. Intra-operatively, the gentle rubbing of the angled laparoscope lens on the liver surface can also be attempted to clear the condensation; this method becomes considerably less successful however, once the liver surface is itself covered with a layer of oil and water from the adjacent cautery. Newer anti-fogging devices have been developed which allows for intra-operative warming and cleansing of the telescope lens by way of a battery-operated docking system, which we have used with some success (Fig. 2).

The first assistant stands on the right side of the patient at approximately the level of the camera assistant, if needed. His/her main purpose for the majority of the operation is to retract the gallbladder over the inferior edge of the liver. His/her grip on the gallbladder should remain still, and should

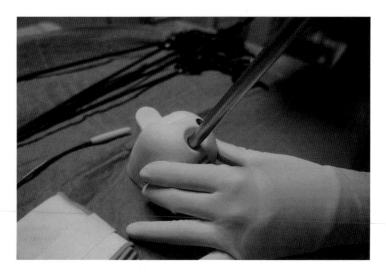

Figure 2.   Intra-operative warming and cleansing of the laparoscope.

only move the gallbladder when directed by the surgeon. Pressing the shaft of the grasping forceps against the patient's body with the left hand, while the right hand grips the instrument handle firmly can attain additional leverage in lifting the gallbladder over the liver. A piece of gauze placed strategically between the instrument port and the patient's skin helps to avoid pressure injury.

Creation of Pneumoperitoneum

The initial incision is made in the peri-umbilical region; depending on surgeon preference, this can be trans-umbilical, supra-umbilical or infra-umbilical. We prefer a 10 mm curved infra-umbilical following the circumference of the navel, for cosmesis and ease of wound closure and dressing. The skin is stretched lightly with the help of the non-dominant hand, and the incision made to breach the dermis (Fig. 3).

The subcutaneous fat, Camper's fascia and Scarpa's fascia are bluntly cleared with a pair of artery forceps. The non-dominant hand maintains an opening in the tissues with its artery forceps' jaws open, while the dominant hand spreads apart deeper layers of tissues in a direction perpendicular to the

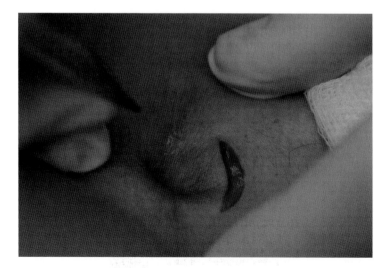

Figure 3.   An infra-umbilical curved incision is made to breach the dermis.

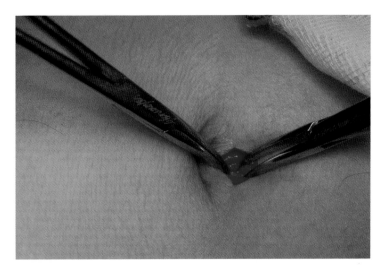

Figure 4. Exposure of the rectus sheath using artery forceps to dissect the overlying fascia.

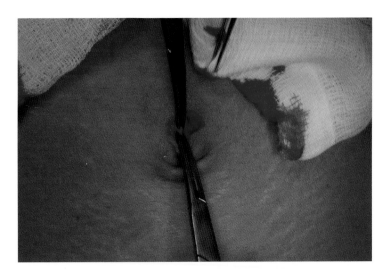

Figure 5. The rectus sheath is grasped on both sides with forceps.

horizontal direction (Fig. 4). Any deviation from a straight-down direction may result in subsequent injury of muscle layers and blood vessels, with irksome bleeding.

The rectus sheath can be recognised by its opalescent white sheen, and is picked up between the two artery forceps (Fig. 5). Using a scalpel, the rectus

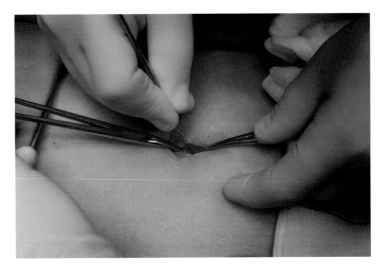

Figure 6. The rectus sheath is then incised with a blade.

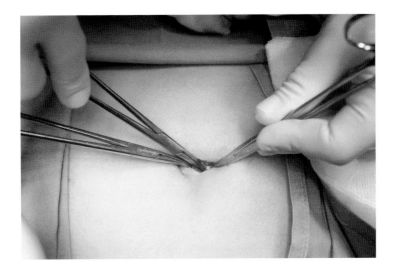

Figure 7. Blunt dissection proceeds gently with forceps.

sheath is incised in the same direction as the skin incision, with the "grittiness" affirming that the rectus sheath is indeed being cut (Fig. 6).

With the two artery forceps holding up the incised rectus sheath on each side, a third artery forceps is now used to bluntly dissect the pre-peritoneal fat and peritoneum layer until the peritoneum is breached (Fig. 7).

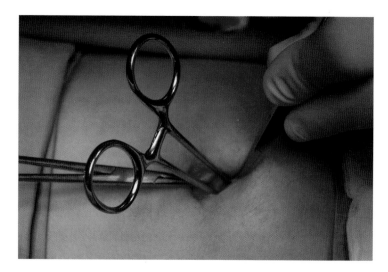

Figure 8. There should be a palpable "give" as the peritoneum is entered, and the entire length of the forceps should be able to slide in without resistance.

The penetration of the peritoneum can be felt as a give, and the smooth insertion of an artery forceps deep into the incision without resistance can be taken as confirmation of entry into the peritoneal cavity (Fig. 8).

The risk of injury to bowel during this entire process is minimal due to the ratcheting up of the abdominal wall by the artery forceps. Anchoring sutures are placed on the rectus sheath where the artery forceps are placed, and the Hassan cannula is inserted into the peritoneal cavity with the help of an introducer rod (Fig. 9).

The anchoring sutures are then wound around the Hassan port to secure it in place and avoid accidental dislodgment during the operation (Fig. 10). Subsequently, carbon dioxide is introduced via the Hassan cannula to insufflate the abdomen.

The laparoscope is inserted via the Hassan cannula to do an initial diagnostic laparoscopic examination. This entails not only inspecting the right upper abdominal region for associated inflammation, but also looking out for other incidental intra-abdominal pathology not suspected pre-operatively. These include inguinal hernias, fatty liver, endometriosis, and the rare malignancy.

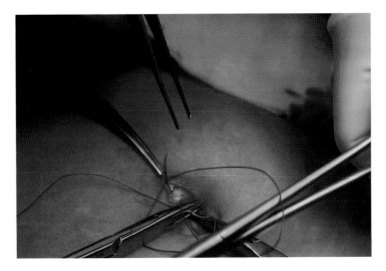

Figure 9. Anchoring sutures are then placed through the fascia.

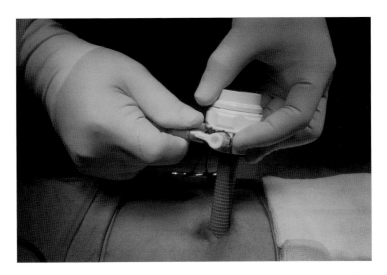

Figure 10. The umbilical port is inserted and secured with sutures, following which the pneumoperitoneum is created.

Ports Placement

Three ports are usually placed in the subcostal area. The first port is inserted just to the right of the falciform ligament. The second port is placed approximately 2 cm below the right costal margin in line with the

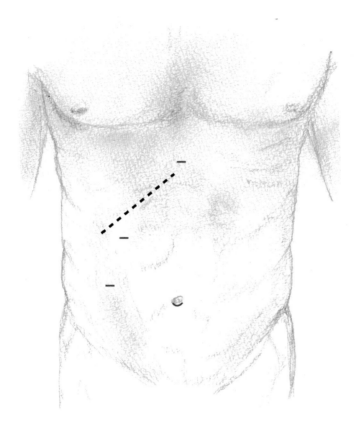

Figure 11. Diagram showing the usual incision sites. Marked in red are the usual laparoscopic incisions. Dotted in black is the incision site of a conventional open cholecystectomy.

gallbladder. The third and most lateral port is placed approximately 2 cm below the costal margin in the anterior axillary line (Fig. 11). A good working practice would be to palpate the intended point of entry into the peritoneal cavity with the index finger to gauge and adjust the incision site. All ports must be placed under direct vision, to avoid inadvertent injury to organs (Fig. 12).

The initial direction of pressure when inserting the ports should be perpendicular to the skin surface, but angled towards the operative site after the fascia has been breached and just before penetrating the peritoneum (Fig. 13). This will allow for minimal tissue trauma, secure port placement, and an ergonomically advantageous working port positions. The size of the ports may differ between

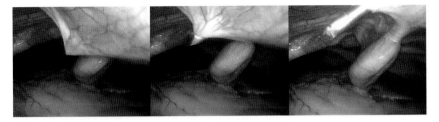

Figure 12. Insertion of ports under direct vision. As the trocar begins to breach the peritoneum, the surgeon eases the pressure exerted to prevent accidental visceral injury. As the trocar tip enters the peritoneal cavity, it is advanced slightly further in before the removal of the trocar, leaving the port in place.

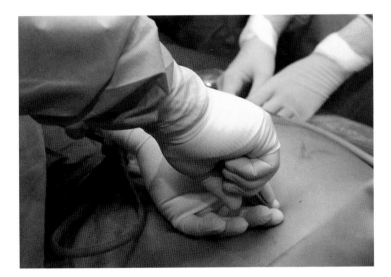

Figure 13. Place the base of the port against your palm and grasp the rest of the port with your index finger aligned along the shaft. With a twisting motion, advance the port slowly through the incision until the peritoneum is breached before removing the trocar. The index finger along the shaft is pressed upon the abdomen during the insertion process, and serves to prevent the port from over-extending into the peritoneal cavity.

surgeons, but are usually 5–10 mm in size. The authors' preference is for the xiphoid port to be 5 mm in size, while the other two subcostal ports 3 mm or 5 mm in size, depending on the expected complexity of the case (Fig. 14).

On occasion, the gallbladder is not readily visible upon initial laparoscopic examination. After insertion of the 5 mm xiphoid port, a grasper can

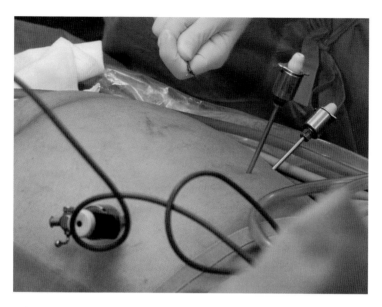

Figure 14.   Placement of three subcostal ports completed (view from patient's left shoulder).

then be used to retract the surrounding omentum and bowel away to reveal the gallbladder. The presence, or absence of inflammation and/or adhesions can then guide the surgeon's port size choices for the remaining two ports.

The first and second ports are used as the working ports, through which the surgeon inserts laparoscopic instruments for the manipulation and dissection of the gallbladder. The third port is handled by the assistant, and is used to grasp the gallbladder fundus and retract it over the inferior edge of the liver. This allows for better exposure and dissection of Calot's triangle. Some surgeons advocate laparoscopic cholecystectomy without this third port, citing less pain and no difference in operating times and complications whilst using only the two working ports. We prefer to use the conventional three working ports method, as we feel that exposure of Calot's triangle provided by the lifting of the gallbladder by the third working port makes the operation much safer and efficient.

Dissection and Resection

Following the insertion of the ports, the authors routinely insert gauze strips via the Hassan cannula, even for the most routine and simple of cases. The

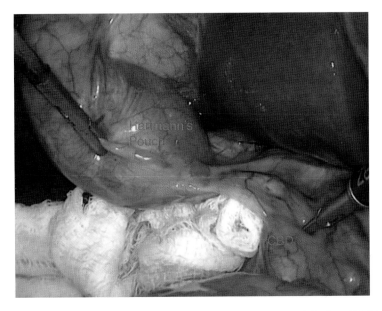

Figure 15. Pre-dissection with gauze strips inserted. The common bile duct (CBD) and Hartmann's pouch can be clearly appreciated here.

minimum number of gauze strips used is three, with more being inserted based on the complexity of the case (Fig. 15).

The key stages of the procedure are listed as how the authors would perform a routine laparoscopic cholecystectomy, but individual cases need not follow this particular sequence. Indeed, it is probably more often that the authors deviate from the below mentioned sequence than follow it exactly depending on the unique circumstances presented in different patients. The reader is likewise encouraged to be flexible and adapt the operation to the anatomical variations he/she may encounter, and challenges that may arise from each specific case.

Calot's triangle is the space bound superiorly by the inferior edge of the liver, medially by the common hepatic duct, and inferiorly by the cystic duct. The cystic artery is usually found in the triangle. Careful dissection and exposure of the triangle gives the surgeon the "critical view". The dissection of the areolar tissue that separates the cystic duct from the inferior liver plate is crucial to obtain this critical view. There is no need for dissection to the junction of the cystic artery and the common bile duct, as long as the critical view can be ascertained.

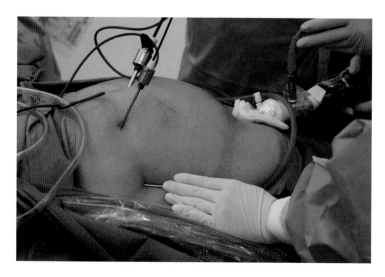

Figure 16. Extra-corporeal view of the first assistant providing cephalic retraction of the gallbladder. The use of the left hand to flatten the instrument shaft against the abdominal surface allows the instrument to be pushed further up above the costal margin to provide for increased retraction of the gallbladder.

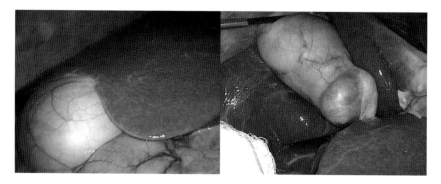

Figure 17. The left image shows the gallbladder prior to retraction. The gallbladder is grasped at its fundus and retracted by the first assistant over the liver edge, exposing the Hartmann's pouch in the right image.

The first assistant first retracts the gallbladder in the cephalad direction over the liver edge (Figs. 16 and 17). This is usually straightforward, and best achieved by grasping the gallbladder fundus. However, there are cases where a distended gallbladder (or mucocele of the gallbladder) makes grasping and retraction a challenge. In such cases, it is advisable to aspirate the gallbladder, thereby collapsing it and making it much easier to grasp (Fig. 18). If there is persistent bile leakage from the aspiration puncture site of the gallbladder, it is preferable to grasp the gallbladder at the puncture site during retraction to prevent excess spillage of bile.

The approximate junction of the cystic duct and common bile duct is first identified through the hepatoduodenal ligament, made clearer by pulling the gallbladder laterally with the left working hand. The dissection starts closer to the neck of the gallbladder rather than the cystic duct-common bile duct junction, to reduce the risk of accidental thermal injury to the common bile duct (Fig. 19).

The authors use a "dolphin-nosed" grasper with the right working hand to perform dissection with monopolar cautery, allowing for minute amounts of tissue to be dissected at a time. A small amount of tissue is grasped and lifted off the underlying vital structures, following which cautery is applied, and the cauterised tissue pulled gently off in a sideways direction (Fig. 20). Holding the gauze strip(s) and rubbing the tissue in an up-and-down manner performs blunt dissection remarkably well. In cases where irrigation is required, the tip of the suction apparatus can also work well as a blunt dissector in combination with a stream of warm saline.

Through a combination of cautery and blunt dissection, Calot's triangle can usually be easily cleared of tissue. Placing a gauze strip behind Calot's triangle whilst dissecting anteriorly backwards can be a great aid in differentiating between the cystic duct, cystic artery and non-vital fatty tissue. Calot's triangle should ideally be cleared to the extent that the bare inferior surface of the liver can be visualised, and near to the junction of the cystic duct and common bile duct (Fig. 21). This amount of meticulous dissection will allow for the identification of aberrant anatomy, and prevent accidental ligation and damage to a replaced right hepatic artery, as an example.

The lymph node known as Cloquet's node points to the site of the cystic artery. The cystic duct is usually located below the artery as part of the boundary of Calot's triangle. Preferably, the path of the cystic duct from the gallbladder neck to the common bile duct should be readily appreciable (Fig. 22).

Gallstones entrapped within the cystic duct or gallbladder neck can be easily palpated with the forceps, and attempts should be made to gently milk them back into the gallbladder prior to ligation of the duct (Fig. 23).

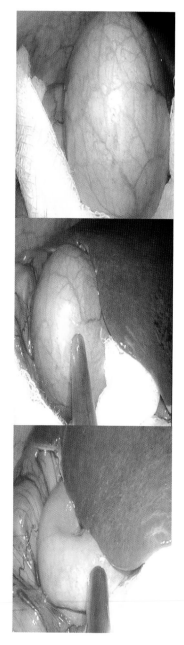

Figure 18.   Sequential images showing a heavily distended gallbladder being aspirated. The gallbladder can then be retracted cephalad easily.

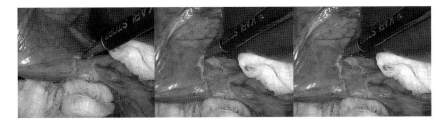

Figure 19. The initial dissection can be carried out further away from the common bile duct, along the plane between the liver and the gallbladder.

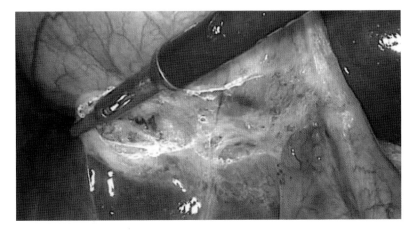

Figure 20. Dissection being carried out posteriorly between the gallbladder and liver, using the dolphin-nosed forceps.

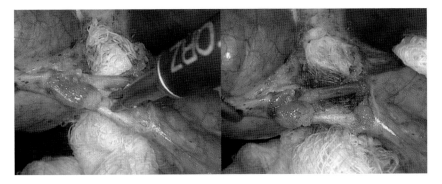

Figure 21. Areolar tissue can be dissected off carefully until the cystic artery (superior) and cystic duct (inferior) are clearly identified. The gauze strips placed behind the structures provide contrast, soak up liquid debris and prevent thermal injury to adjacent structures.

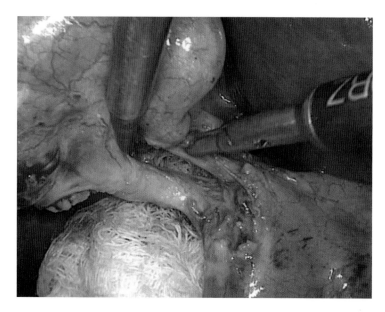

Figure 22. By inserting the left-hand instrument into the aperture between the cystic artery and cystic duct, additional space is created for safer dissection.

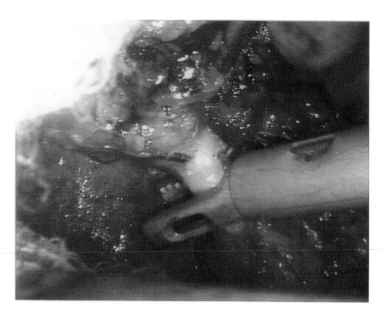

Figure 23. A stone palpated in the cystic duct is milked back to the gallbladder before ligation and transection.

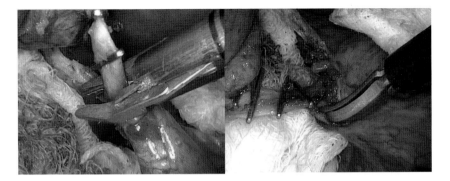

Figure 24. Ensure the tips of the clip applicator can be seen before deploying any clips to prevent including other structures inadvertently. Laparoscopic scissors are then used to divide the ligated cystic artery and cystic duct.

The cystic duct is ligated with the placement of clips, and transected with scissors (Figs. 24 and 25). In cases where the cystic duct is oedematous or distended and cannot be fully secured with clips, ties can be secured around the cystic duct either intracorporeally or extracorporeally based on surgeon's preference (Fig. 26). In difficult cases, an alternative would be to transect the cystic duct first, then suture ligate the stump (Fig. 27).

The cystic artery can similarly be ligated and transected, or electro-coagulated in cases where the artery is deemed to be small enough. The cut edge of the cystic duct should be inspected to confirm that that there is undeniably only one lumen, and not two lumens (the latter would suggest the common bile duct has been erroneously ligated with the cystic duct, and a complex repair procedure is in order).

The authors routinely use a disposable automated metal clip applier, although re-usable metal clip appliers are also commonly used. Advanced energy sources are not part of our usual armamentarium for laparoscopic cholecystectomy. In our experience, the careful and accurate use of monopolar cautery usually suffices for all dissecting and haemostatic purposes.

The rest of the procedure involves the dissection of the gallbladder off the liver with electro-coagulation (Figs. 28 and 29). We favour the use of the hook diathermy for this part of the operation. Its fine angled tip allows for pinpoint cautery and hooking of tissue strands, or a broader field of cautery using the heel of the hook when needed. The mist created by the cautery may

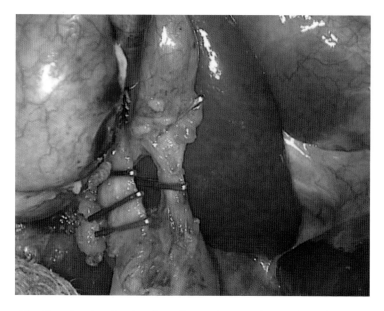

Figure 25. Posterior view showing three clips on the cystic duct and two clips on the cystic artery. Two clips and one clip will be left on the cystic duct stump and cystic artery stump respectively post-operatively. This is to aid the identification of the structures if complications arise and a re-operation is required.

be quite significant, and opening the valve on one of the ports other than the Hassan port can help in its dissipation. In cases where the inflammation blurs the plane between the gallbladder and liver, it is advisable to stick closer to the side of the gallbladder; perforation of the gallbladder is relatively easy to remedy, while uncontrolled bleeding from the liver parenchyma may be catastrophic.

Specimen Retrieval, Irrigation and Drains

There exists a range of commercial retrieval devices that are meant to aid the fuss-free retrieval of the gallbladder from the abdomen. Most of their pouches are made from a tough, slightly elastic plastic material, which can contain the gallbladder and resist tearing. These pouches usually contain a spring-loaded purse-string mechanism that prevents spillage of the pouch's contents.

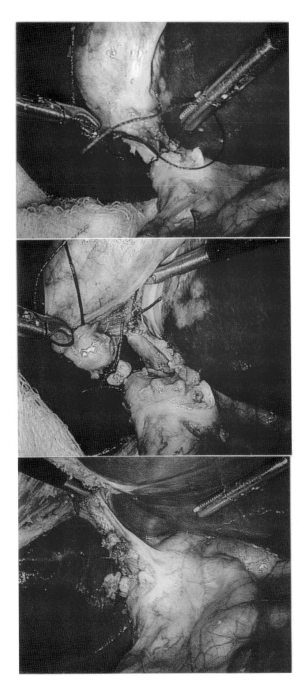

Figure 26. Intracorporeal suture ligation of the cystic duct. The cystic duct is then transected between the ties.

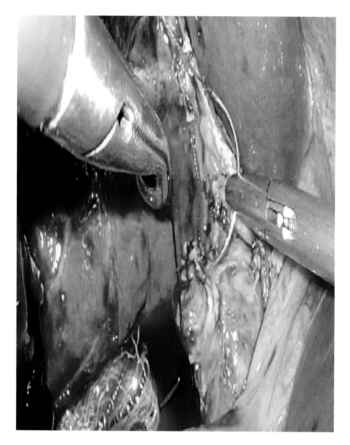

Figure 27.   Suture ligation of a cystic duct stump in a case of acute cholecystitis, where the inflammation caused reactive edema of the cystic duct.

The retrieval devices are sized to fit through a 10 mm port, namely the peri-umbilical port used for the laparoscope for the majority of the operation. This part of the operation hence normally requires the insertion of the laparoscope through the xiphoid port. The same laparoscope can be used if the medial most subcostal port was 10 mm in size, otherwise the laparoscope will have to be changed to a 5 mm sized one.

The authors currently prefer to use a simple self-made plastic pouch with a purse-string suture and sliding knot incorporated at its opening. The pouch is inserted via the 10 mm peri-umbilical port, with the end of the suture remaining outside the body. The laparoscope can be reinserted via the same

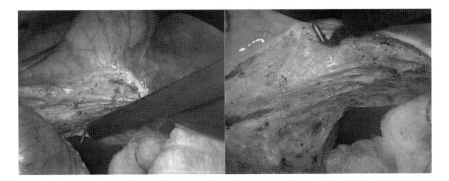

Figure 28. Use of the hook diathermy for dissection of the gallbladder off the liver. The first assistant and left hand of the surgeon provides the traction needed for a clean dissection through the avascular plane between the gallbladder and liver.

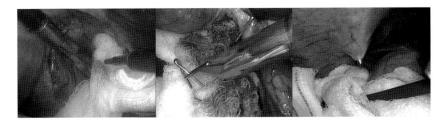

Figure 29. The uses of gauze strips are numerous and we consider them an indispensable part of the operation. The left image depicts the use of gauze strips as a blunt dissector at Calot's triangle. The centre image illustrates how it soaks up liquid debris from the dissection process, as well as being an effective depot for other solid debris like misfired clips. The right image demonstrates how it allows for safe retraction of tissues, in this case the shielding of the colon during insertion of the subcostal ports.

10 mm Hassan cannula, sliding in alongside the suture within the port. The bag is positioned above the liver surface and laid open to receive the gallbladder and gauze strips. Simultaneously holding onto the sliding knot and pulling on the suture outside the body closes the pouch (Figs. 30 and 31).

Routine irrigation after an uncomplicated cholecystectomy is not needed. However, when there is bile spillage or severe inflammation, then irrigation with normal saline is indicated.

Irrigation and suction is not limited to the end of the operation and should be done as and when the need arises. Some argue that irrigation may increase the risk of peritoneal contamination by allowing spread of the

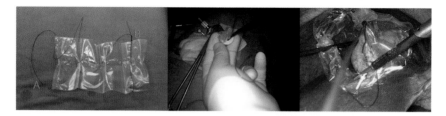

Figure 30. The plastic pouch in the left image has a purse-string suture enclosing its opening. To close the pouch, (A) is pulled extracorporeally while (B) is grasped unto intracorporeally simultaneously. It is inserted via the 10 mm umbilical port as shown in the centre image. Subsequently, it is placed over the liver surface for the collection of the specimen, gauze strips, and other debris.

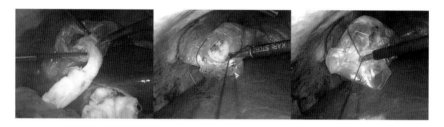

Figure 31. After all specimens and debris have been inserted into the pouch, the knot of the purse-string suture is grasped, and the suture end lying extra-corporeally is pulled upon, thus closing the purse-string suture.

pollutants intra-operatively. So long as the subphrenic and subhepatic spaces, gallbladder bed, and paracolic gutters are carefully suctioned prior to the end of the operation, the risk of a post-operative collection is negligible (Fig. 32).

Routine drain placements are not indicated. But in situations where the surgeon feels the risk of a post-operative collection is significant, drains can then be placed. The common locations include the subphrenic space, gallbladder bed, Morrison's pouch, and right paracolic gutter (Fig. 33).

These drains are usually small-bored, and connected to a closed suction system (Fig. 34). Up to three drains can be placed, usually via the subcostal ports. Their eventual removal is decided based on clinical judgment by the surgeon.

The contents of the retrieval pouch are then removed via the peri-umbilical incision. A pair of sponge forceps can be used to stretch out the fascia opening to aid in specimen removal. The closed jaws of the sponge forceps

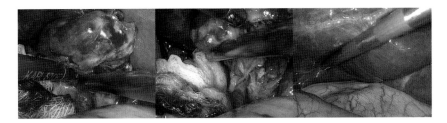

Figure 32. The left image illustrates the use of irrigation and the suction apparatus as a dissecting tool for an inflamed gallbladder. The centre image depicts irrigation and suction in combination with gauze strips; suctioning upon the gauze strips ensures that the suctioning process does not injure adjacent structures like the omentum and colon. The aim is for the operative field to be as spotless as possible, like the Morrison's pouch shown in the right image post-irrigation.

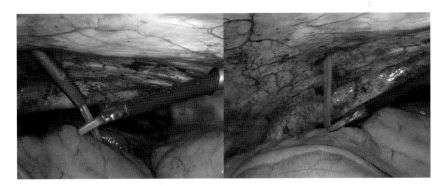

Figure 33. The drain is inserted via one of the subcostal ports, and put in position by a pair of forceps. The port is then removed, as the drain is held in placed. The drain is usually secured by means of a suture on the abdominal wall.

are placed at the fascia opening. The jaws are then opened in a smooth but firm manner to stretch out the aponeurotic fibres. The jaws of the forceps are then rotated 90°, and the process repeated a few times till a satisfactory result is achieved.

The gallbladder may have to be emptied of its bile in some cases before removal. The wall of the gallbladder is grasped at two points with artery forceps, and the gallbladder is entered with a pair or sharp scissors, with a suction apparatus on standby to prevent bile spillage. Once the gallbladder is entered, the suction apparatus is inserted into the opening and the bile suctioned out. Gallstones *in situ* may also hinder the extraction of the gallbladder. Gallstones may then need to be patiently crushed or scooped out with specially designed stone forceps. In cases of a thickened and oedematous gallbladder, the gallbladder may have to be removed piecemeal.

Throughout the entire process of removing the contents of the retrieval bag, it is a good habit to surround the opening of the bag with a few pieces of gauze. This is meant to provide a physical barrier between potential spillage from the bag and the peri-umbilical wound (Figs. 34–37). A renegade gallstone or runaway stream of bile contaminating the wound leads to

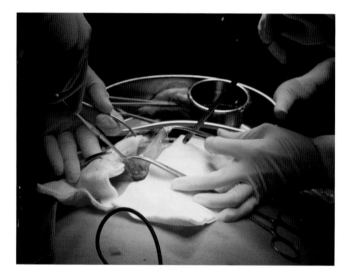

Figure 34. Hold the pouch open by way of four artery forceps, and use a sponge forceps to stretch out the incision if needed. The opening of the bag is surrounded by gauze to prevent bile spillage onto the wound. A suction device and kidney dish to hold instruments and debris are readily at hand.

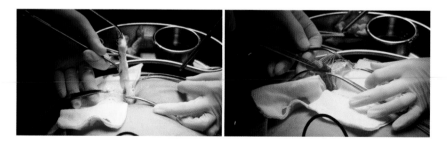

Figure 35. Gauze strips and the gallbladder are subsequently removed with forceps.

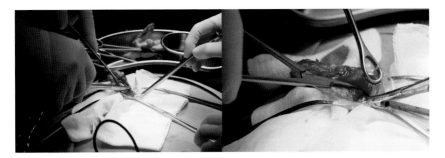

Figure 36. If the gallbladder is unable to be removed whole, it is then incised with scissors and the bile suctioned. Gallstones are usually the cause precluding the whole removal of gallbladders.

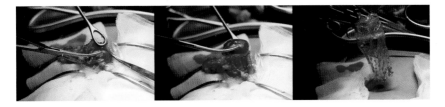

Figure 37. The culpable gallstone is removed, and the gallbladder is removed without further incident. Ensure that the pouch is intact upon removal.

increased risk of wound infection and breakdown, and this simple practice helps mitigate the risk. When inserting instruments into the bag to retrieve objects, the amount of force used must be moderated. This avoids the danger of accidentally rupturing the bag and allowing its contents to fall back into the peritoneal cavity.

Fascia and Wound Closure

This portion of the operation is crucial, and requires due care to avoid an iatrogenic hernia. Diligence with regards to wound irrigation may also help decrease the rate of wound infection, especially if there has been spillage of biliary contents intra-operatively. Either copious amounts of normal saline or plain chlorhexidine is sufficient for wound decontamination (Fig. 38).

The anchoring suture, if placed during the initial entry into the peritoneal cavity, now serves to hold up and expose the fascia. There are many

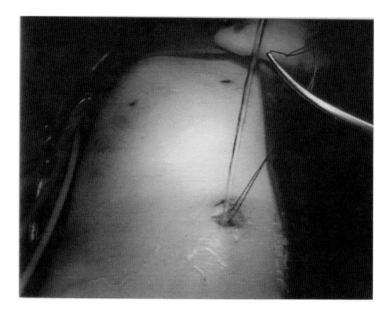

Figure 38. The peri-umbilical incision is routinely irrigated with normal saline to decrease the risk of wound infection. This image illustrates the use of the remnant normal saline meant for intra-operative irrigation of the peritoneal cavity to irrigate the wounds.

different ways surgeons close the fascia, but the underlying principles are the same. The fascia must be included in the stitch, while avoiding muscle. Tension must be firm but not overly tight. The suture used should be absorbable to avoid a foreign body reaction and granuloma formation in the long term.

The authors routinely place a figure-of-eight stitch on either side of the central anchoring suture, ensuring that the corner of the cut fascia has been incorporated. The central anchoring suture is then itself secured, creating a fortified seal of the rectus sheath (Figs. 39 and 40).

The skin can be closed with non-absorbable or absorbable sutures. Non-absorbable monofilament sutures are normally used for simple interrupted or vertical mattress sutures. Braided or monofilament sutures are used for subcuticular closure. We prefer the use of non-absorbable monofilament sutures, which we remove after 5–7 days post-operatively (Figs. 41 and 42).

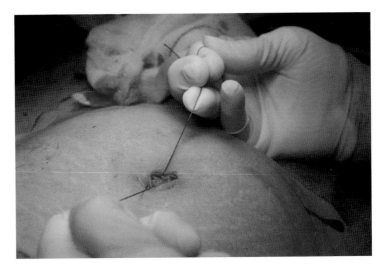

Figure 39. The assistant holds up the anchoring suture that had been placed initially during the Hassan port insertion, exposing the rectus sheath and drawing the abdominal wall away from the peritoneal contents. This makes it easier for the surgeon to place stitches on both sides of the anchoring suture.

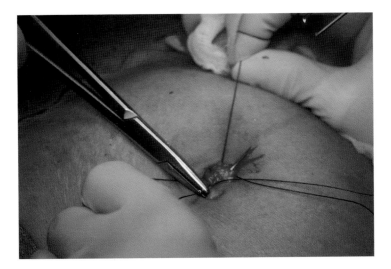

Figure 40. The rectus sheath is elevated by the anchoring suture by the assistant, allowing the surgeon to place two more sutures incorporating the rectus sheath on either side of the anchoring suture.

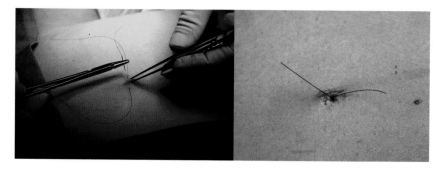

Figure 41. Vertical mattress closure of subcostal port incisions.

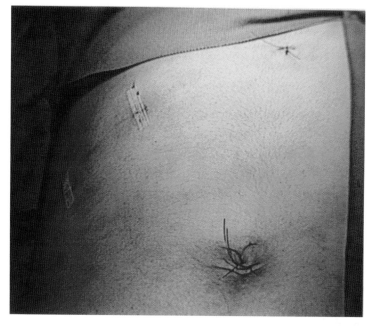

Figure 42. Immediate post-operative view of the incisions.

Needlescopic Laparoscopy

An alternative form of laparoscopic surgery is needlescopic surgery, which essentially utilises smaller diameter laparoscopic instruments to carry out the same procedure (Fig. 43). These needlescopic instruments measure 1–2 mm in diameter, and a 5 mm sized laparoscope is usually used in tandem with the

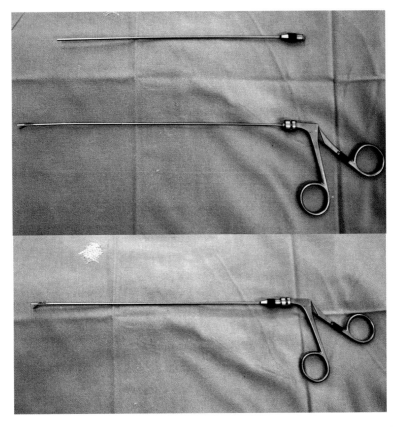

Figure 43. The above image shows the needlescopic grasper before assembly, and the bottom image shows the grasper after assembly.

concept of smaller incisions. As expected, the instruments are more delicate, with reduced grasping ability and require the surgeon to be prudent with the amount of torque and force placed on the instruments. Extra care is especially needed when lifting the gallbladder over the liver with the lateral-most subcostal instrument, as the mechanical stress on the shaft and forcep jaws are the greatest (Figs. 44 and 45).

This approach is reasonable for patients with thin abdominal walls that place less stress on the instrument shafts, and uncomplicated straightforward elective cases in the absence of acute inflammation. Choosing a needlescopic approach initially does not prevent the surgeon from switching to the use of normal sized laparoscopic instruments if the need arises during the operation.

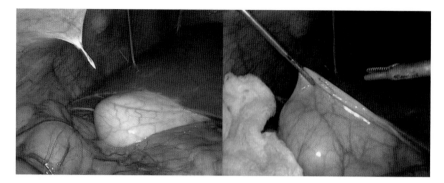

Figure 44.   Left image shows peritoneal entry under direct vision of the needlescopic grasper. The needlescopic instrument is able to grasp non-inflamed, non-oedematous gallbladders, as shown in the right image.

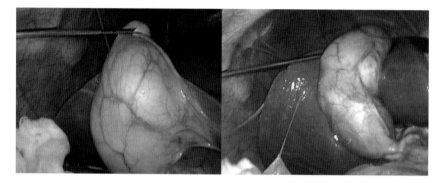

Figure 45.   The left image shows the needlescopic forceps twisting to provide more grip during retraction. Unlike normal laparoscopic instruments where there is a dial at the base of the instrument next to the handle for the twisting of the shaft, a needlescopic instrument needs to be rotated in its entirety as it lacks a rotating dial. The right image shows the liver successfully retracted over the liver edge. The fragile shaft of the needlescopic instrument needs to be flattened manually against the abdominal wall during this process to prevent it from being bent.

Less post-operative pain can be expected with this approach, though recovery time remains similar to routine laparoscopic surgery. With the exception of the peri-umbilical incision used for the laparoscope insertion, other incisions can be sealed with steri-strips.

Post-operative Phase

Post-operative care begins when the patient is wheeled out of the operating room, and does not have a defined end-point. Even after discharge, patients return to the clinic for post-operative follow-up consultations. It is uncommon, but not unheard of, to have patients presenting years after the initial laparoscopic cholecystectomy with issues related to long-term complications.

Post-operative Wound Care

Wounds can be reinforced with steri-strips. Simple waterproof dressing usually suffices for the protection of wounds, and can be removed 24 hours after the operation. Wounds become "water-tight" 24–48 hours after closure, and non-absorbable sutures can routinely be removed within 5–7 days in the absence of any complications.

Superficial wound infection is uncommon after laparoscopic cholecystectomy, and deep-seated wound infections even more so. However any symptoms and signs of wound infection, such as erythema and pain and tenderness, warrants oral antibiotics. A more severe wound infection with pus formation warrant wound opening, packing and intravenous antibiotics. Very rarely does the wound infection progress to necrotising fasciitis, a potentially fatal condition that requires immediate surgical debridement.

Infections that involve the fascia invariably increase the risk of hernia formation. Patients may present months or years later with a bulge of their abdominal wall. Though uncommon, incisional hernias that do occur almost invariably involve the periumbilical incision. The risk of bowel incarceration and strangulation is high due to the narrow neck of the hernia, and should be repaired as early as possible.

In-hospital Care

Whilst in the recovery room, patients experiencing massive haemorrhage can turn haemodynamically unstable, and must be brought back to the operating room for an immediate re-exploration. Other symptoms and signs that would suggest sinister post-operative bleeding include referred shoulder pain, increasing abdominal distension, and large amount of bloody effluent from drains if present. The offending bleed may arise from the cystic artery stump, an accidentally injured right hepatic artery and/or liver parenchyma from inadvertent lacerations. In patients with portal hypertension, bleeding may also arise from the falciform ligament.

For uncomplicated elective cases, patients can usually be discharged within 24 hours after the operation. Patients with incision site pain refractory to prescribed analgesics may need increased dosages before they are confident enough to return home. The return of ambulation and tolerance of oral intake are also required before the patient is allowed home. The return of bowel movements is not routinely used as a threshold for discharge.

Patients who undergo a laparoscopic cholecystectomy for an acutely inflamed gallbladder or empyema will normally be observed past 24 hours. They may require a longer duration of intravenous antibiotics, and usually do not return to oral intake as quickly due to ileus. If drains were placed, they can be removed 2–3 days after the surgery at the surgeon's discretion. Patients need not be kept in hospital until the removal of drains; they can be removed during a scheduled clinic consultation after proper drain care instructions have been dispensed.

In cases where a conversion to an open procedure had to be performed, patients can expect to stay considerably longer. The right subcostal incision, or Kocher's incision, is significantly larger and more painful than laparoscopic incisions due to the amount of severed muscle fibres involved (Fig. 1).

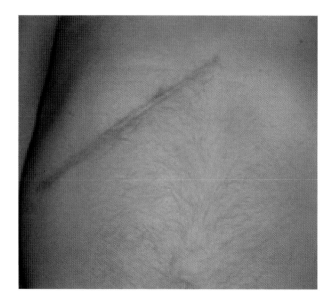

Figure 1.   Scar of a well-healed open cholecystectomy incision.

Analgesic requirements will increase, as will the patients' reluctance to ambulate or breathe deeply. These can lead on to a substantial increased risk of atelectasis, pneumonia, deep vein thrombosis and pulmonary embolism. Active chest and ambulatory physiotherapy, with the possible addition of anticoagulants can help lessen these risks. The criteria for discharge remain the same as for uncomplicated laparoscopic cases, and should be made based on the progress of each individual.

Post-discharge Follow-up

Patients with non-absorbable sutures will usually return to the clinic within 5 days for wound inspection and suture removal (Fig. 2). Patients who are discharged with drains may be given specific follow-up instructions with regards to timing and frequency of follow-up visits. All other patients with an uncomplicated inpatient stay usually return within 2 weeks for a routine visit.

Subsequently, the frequency of repeat consultations is highly variable among patients. This depends on the initial reason for operation, the need

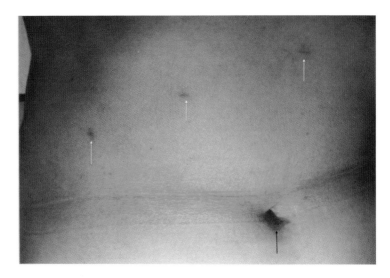

Figure 2. Well-healed incisions of a patient who underwent laparoscopic cholecystectomy, approximately 6 weeks post-operative.

for future surgical or endoscopic intervention, patients' alleviation of symptoms, and patients' comfort and satisfaction. Patients who undergo elective laparoscopic cholecystectomy for benign disease and experience full resolution of their symptoms usually require no more than a second clinic consultation before being discharged from routine follow-up.

Patient can present months to years after the initial operation, with symptoms and signs suggestive of obstruction or infection of the biliary tree. Strictures of the biliary tree related to the inflammation or caused by the operation is not uncommon. Common bile duct stones, whether retained from the last operation, or primarily formed in the common bile duct, also do arise occasionally. A full review of the patient's previous radiological studies and surgical operative notes are warranted, enabling potential complications to be explored.

Complications

Laparoscopic cholecystectomy is an extremely safe procedure with major morbidity occurring in less than 5% of patients, and with a mortality rate of less than 0.5%. However, complications do exist and range from simple non-life threatening to catastrophic events.

General Anaesthesia

The risk of undergoing general anaesthesia is dependent heavily on the patient's co-morbidities, age and pre-operative physiological status. The following list of complications is not exhaustive:

- Acute myocardial ischaemia
- Cerebrovascular accident/transient ischaemic attack
- Pneumonia/atelactasis
- Deep vein thrombosis/pulmonary embolism
- Oral-buccal injury (during intubation)

Injury from Trocar/Veress Needle Insertion

In the process of creating the pneumoperitoneum required for laparoscopic surgery via the open Hassan method or Veress needle insertion, injury to organs or blood vessels can occur. Trocars required for the insertion of laparoscopic instruments can also cause such injuries, and incidence rates range from 0.05–0.1% of all laparoscopic cases.

In the event of bowel injury, lacerations can be sutured laparoscopically. Uncontrollable haemorrhage or inability to repair bowel injuries laparoscopically merits a conversion to open surgery for the prevention of further morbidity.

Haemorrhage

Massive bleeding during trocar insertion is rare but may occur when retroperitoneal vessels such as the aorta and vena cava are lacerated. These injuries can be lethal, and hypotension or a rapidly developing retroperitoneal haematoma is an indication for immediate laparotomy.

Excessive bleeding can occur within Calot's triangle or from the liver bed during dissection (Fig. 1). Careful identification of bleeding points and/or vessels is crucial before diathermy or haemostatic clips are applied. Topical haemostatic agents are also available, and topical pressure is a great aide. Argon plasma coagulator (APC) can serve as a tool in states of uncontrollable oozing, with conversion to laparotomy when all laparoscopic attempts at haemostasis have failed.

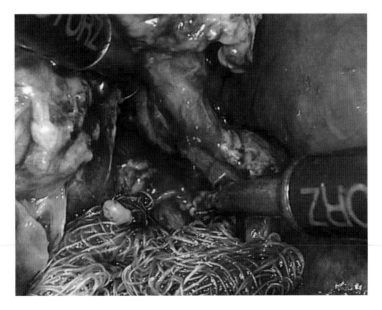

Figure 1. Bleeding during dissection of Calot's triangle. This bleeding was stopped with the use of the dolphin-nosed forceps with diathermy.

Common Bile Duct Injury

The risk of common bile duct injury has been found to be slightly higher in laparoscopic cholecystectomy as compared to the open method, likely due to problems with visualisation. This ranks as the most dreaded of all complications (Fig. 2). Major factors related to the risk of this complication are aberrant anatomy, presence of inflammation, adhesions and severe fibrosis.

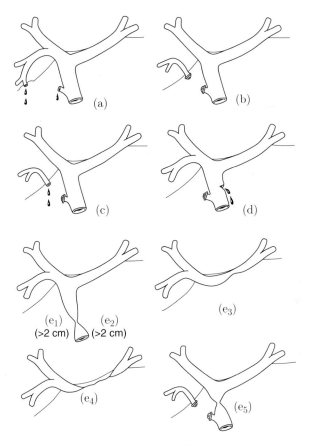

Figure 2. Strasberg-Bismuth classification of bile duct injuries. (a) Cystic duct leaks from small ducts in liver bed. (b) Occlusion of part of the biliary tree typically clipped and divided right hepatic ducts. (c) Transection (but not ligation) of the aberrant right hepatic ducts. (d) Lateral injuries to major bile ducts. (e_1) Common hepatic duct division, >2 cm from bifurcation. (e_2) Common hepatic duct division, <2 cm from bifurcation. (e_3) Common bile duct division at bifurcation. (e_4) Hilar stricture, involvement of confluence and loss of communication between right and left hepatic duct. (e_5) Involvement of aberrant right hepatic duct alone or with concomitant stricture of common hepatic duct.

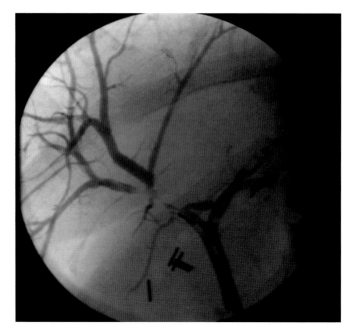

Figure 3. ERCP image showing bile duct injury and stricture post-laparoscopic cholecystectomy.

The presentation and management of common bile duct injuries depend on whether it is diagnosed intra-operatively, or discovered post-operatively. Post-operative presentation can occur either with delayed onset approximately 3–8 days later, or late-onset weeks to months later.

If discovered intra-operatively, management can range from simple laproscopic repair over a T-tube, or construction of a biliary-enteric anastomosis based on the severity of the injury. Delayed presentations usually give rise to symptoms due to bile leaks, and management may require post-operative radiological studies, endoscopic and percutaneous interventions, or even repeat surgeries (Figs. 3–6). Late-onset presentations are usually due to strictures of the bile duct and require endoscopic or surgical intervention to maintain patency of the biliary drainage system.

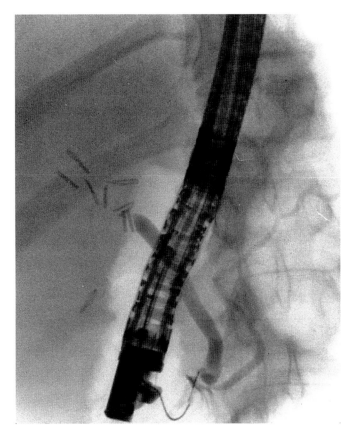

Figure 4. ERCP image post-cholecystectomy, showing multiple clips in the gallbladder bed and a distinct cut-off, depicting ligation of the common bile duct.

Hollow Viscus Injury

In cases of multiple adhesions or acute severe inflammatory conditions of the gallbladder, it is not infrequent for adjacent gastrointestinal structures such as the stomach, duodenum, or colon to be adhered closely to the gallbladder. During particularly difficult portions of the dissection process, these structures may be unintentionally injured. Inadvertent perforation or serosal tears of hollow viscus is a major intra-operative complication that needs to be recognised early.

The decision on whether to repair the injury first, or complete the cholecystectomy depends on the magnitude of injury. If only serosal damage was

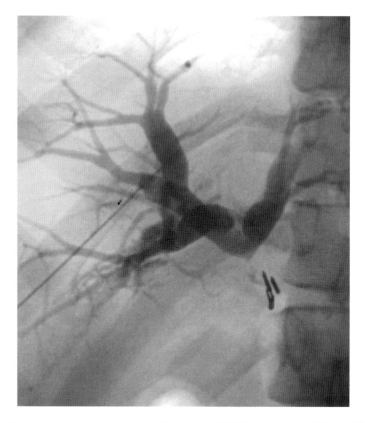

Figure 5. Percutaneous transhepatic cholangiogram (PTC) image showing Type e_2 bile duct injury post-laparoscopic cholecystectomy.

inflicted, then repair can usually be left till the end of the procedure. However, full-thickness perforations with active leakage of enteric material require that the defect be mended immediately to present peritoneal contamination. With sound laparoscopic suturing technique, most injuries can be repaired laparoscopically (Fig. 7).

Wound Infection

Cholecystectomy is considered a clean-contaminated operation, and wound infection rates range from 2–5%, although the infection rate in laparoscopic cholecystectomy is considerably lower. The management of a superficial

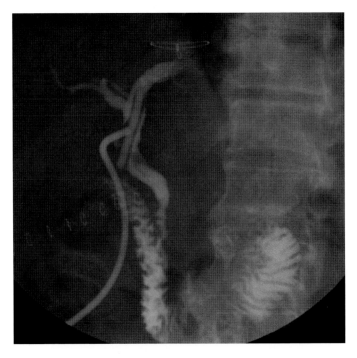

Figure 6. T-tube cholangiogram 2 weeks after a patient had suffered a common bile duct injury, requiring open conversion, and simple repair over a T-tube.

wound infection is the removal of skin staple or sutures to allow simple drainage and dressing, enabling the wound to heal by secondary intention. In rare cases where the wound infection is more deep-seated and involves the fascia, the patient may be acutely ill and require surgical revision of the wound and high-dose intravenous antibiotics. Rarely, the dreaded complication of necrotising fasciitis involving the abdominal wall can occur due to the presence of anaerobic, enteric and commensal bacteria. These can be life threatening and require immediate surgical debridement of all infected tissue.

Post-operative Intra-abdominal Collections

This is usually diagnosed within a week post-operatively, with symptoms of fever and diaphragmatic irritation. The most common areas for post-operative collections are Morrison's pouch or the right sub-diaphragmatic

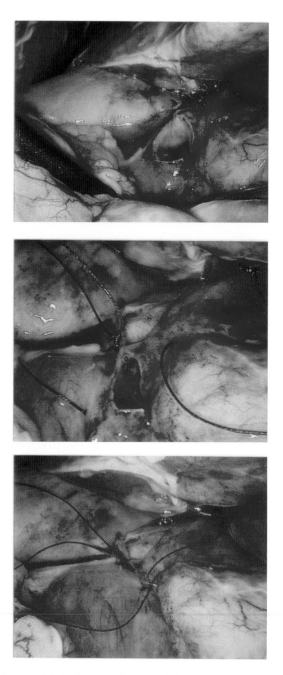

Figure 7. Inadvertent full-thickness perforation of the stomach during laparoscopic chole-cystectomy for acute cholecystitis. The defect was repaired with interrupted absorbable sutures intracorporeally.

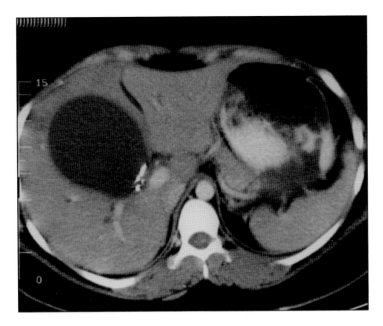

Figure 8. Post-operative biloma likely secondary to cystic duct stump leak.

space. The risk of this complication is increased in acute inflammatory conditions and inadequate irrigation and suction following bile spillage during the operation.

These are diagnosed via radiological means when clinical suspicion is high (Fig. 8). Patients often have persistent fever, tachycardia, raised inflammatory markers and tenderness over the upper abdomen. Depending on the size, location, and sterility of the collection(s), management can range from observation, simple percutaneous drainage, or laparoscopic irrigation. Full laparotomy is rarely required for loculated, infected collections, which are refractory to the above methods.

Ileus

Post-operative ileus occurs more often after open surgery, and when excessive manipulation of the bowel is performed during surgery. Intra-operative anaesthetics and post-operative analgesics also contribute to its occurrence. This complication is fairly rare in laparoscopic cholecystectomy due to the

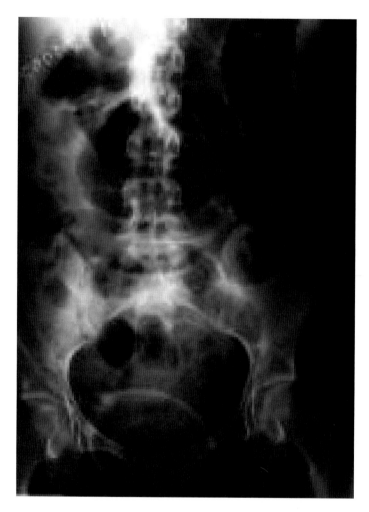

Figure 9. Post-operative ileus in a patient who underwent laparoscopic converted to open cholecystectomy. Note the dilation of both small and large bowel with no transition point.

minimal exposure of bowel to atmospheric air and manipulation. However, it can be substantial in patients who have had severe inflammatory gallstone-related complications, such as gallbladder empyema, gangrenous cholecystitis, cholangitis, and pancreatitis (Fig. 9).

Management usually involves nothing more than ambulation, removal of any possible offending medication and reassurance.

Post-cholecystectomy Syndrome

This represents a spectrum of vague abdominal symptoms, which reflect a myriad of occult gastrointestinal conditions that are not alleviated by chole-cystectomy. These include upper abdominal pain, flatulence, bloating, and dyspepsia. Patients may feel that their symptoms have not improved after surgery, or have even worsened to an extent.

Most commonly, this syndrome is due to dietary indiscretion, with patients consuming too much fatty food than they can tolerate after surgery. This is usually relieved with lifestyle and dietary advice. However, conditions that may require further investigations and treatment include sphincter of Oddi dysfunction, retained common bile duct stones or inflammation of the cystic duct remnant. In addition, stones in a remnant cystic duct or residual gallbladder following a subtotal cholecystectomy can also be a source of recurrent problems. These may require separate endoscopic or operative procedures to fix the underlying issue.

3D Laparoscopic Surgery for Cholecystectomy

Two-dimensional laparoscopy has some disadvantages in terms of visualisation. Surgeons will need secondary spatial cues such as shadows and motion parallax to overcome the inherent limitations of the projected image; the instruments are aligned in a triangulation to allow easy access and visualisation during dissection and suturing. This however takes years of experience to master and still causes considerable mental strain even in the most experienced of surgeons when parallax error occurs.

Three-dimensional (3D) laparoscopic systems were first introduced in the mid-1990s, but failed to gain widespread acceptance due to poor image quality, inadequate lighting and bulky 3D glasses. The camera systems then were heavy and often unwieldy.

Recent advances in the field, however, overcame these issues and 3D laparoscopic surgery is becoming commonplace especially in operative procedures where precision is a premium. Current eyewear is less bulky, and its shape has improved ergonomically to lessen the stress upon on the eyes and face of its users (Figs. 1 and 2).

The technology behind providing a 3D laparoscopic image is fairly straightforward. Located at the distal end of the laparoscope are two high-resolution charge-coupled device (CCD) image sensors, which provide left and right images. These two image signals are then processed by a special-purpose video system to generate a high-resolution 3D image. The image is

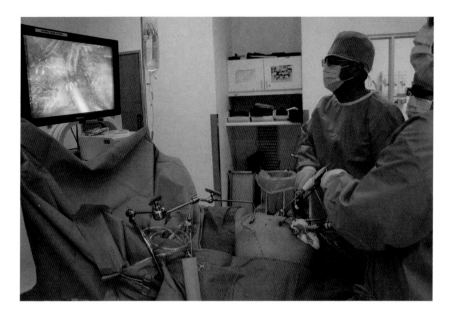

Figure 1.   Surgeons and assistants wear 3D eyeglasses while looking at special 3D projection screens.

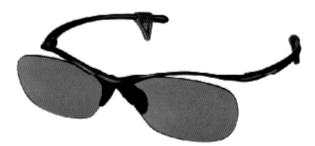

Figure 2.   An example of modern, lightweight 3D glasses. (Copyright© 2014 Olympus. All rights reserved. Used with permission of Olympus.)

then projected on a 3D monitor with 3D glasses used by the surgeons and assistants to create the final realistic image. Clip-on lenses too are readily available for wearers of prescription glasses.

As with current 2D laparoscopic systems, there are also 3D laparoscopes that have a deflectable tip, allowing up to 100° of motion in four directions. This flexibility to view the surgical field from any angle allows the camera assistant to make the most of the limited space in technically demanding procedures; this function is especially useful in a single-port laparoscopic surgery. The visualisation is enhanced even in narrow spaces where access is difficult.

The authors feel that 3D laparoscopy holds the most promise for the advancement of not only laparoscopic cholecystectomy, but for the myriad of surgical procedures now performed endoscopically. Once the surgeon and his surgical team get accustomed to the 3D images, which admittedly may require a period of adjustment initially, the precise level of tissue plane recognition and dissection allowed by the 3D images is unparalleled.

In 3D laparoscopy, there is a minute but perceptible 1–2 mm space, which we dub "the third dimensional space" that is the key to tissue dissection. It is this third-dimensional space that allows surgeons to differentiate between tissue planes for safe, faster and more precise dissection (Fig. 3). This spatial differential is what all future 3D camera systems will seek to exploit in order to bring the tissues to life for the surgical team. The ability to visualise depth and breadth during dissection is unequalled and allows for safer tissue handling during electrocautery. Once this 3D tissue plane is identified,

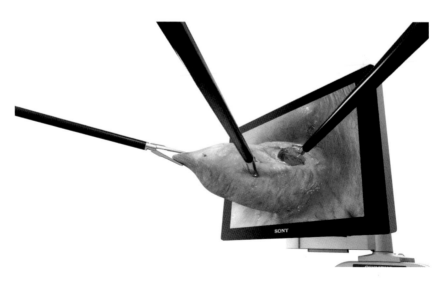

Figure 3. Illustration of the three-dimensional feel of 3D laparoscopy. (Copyright© 2014 Olympus. All rights reserved. Used with permission of Olympus.)

the ability to achieve haemostasis and to proceed in tissue dissection is achievable even under the most challenging of circumstances.

Current 3D camera systems, though excellent, still allow room for improvement. The authors predict the advent of systems, which will allow for the appreciation of 3D images without the use of 3D lenses. With further advancement, these images will be visible from an almost 180° wide angle. This will eventually replace current robotic systems in terms of superiority in suturing and tissue handling, and will pave the way for hand-held robotic instrumentation.

Single Incision Laparoscopic Surgery for Cholecystectomy

Introduced towards the end of the last millennium, single incision laparoscopic surgery for cholecystectomy lacked popularity initially due to a lack of proper instrumentation. However, with the technological strides that have taken place in this field, it now has widespread acceptance as an alternative method to the routine laparoscopic cholecystectomy for selected cases.

This method involves the use of a specialised port system to be inserted via a slightly larger 20 mm peri-umbilical incision, capable of accommodating two or more laparoscopic instruments and a laparoscope. The exact size and number of instruments allowed differ slightly between models. Different commercial brands offer gel-based, balloon-based, or rubber-based models in order to secure the port system to the abdominal wall during the operation (Figs 1 and 2). These port systems are usually single-use and disposable.

Some surgeons have introduced ingenious methods of single incision laparoscopic cholecystectomy in lieu of the commercial port systems. One method is to make multiple adjacent entry sites in the fascia with the same periumbilical skin incision, in a "Mickey Mouse" configuration (Fig. 3). The ports used would need to be short and low profiled in order to avoid clashing with one another. Another involves inserting a sterile glove into the fascia

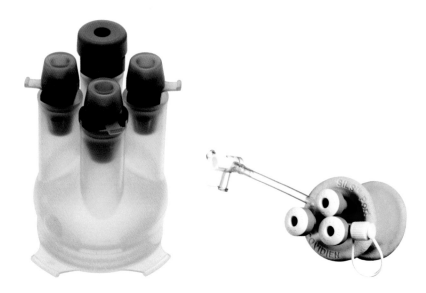

Figure 1. Commercially available single port systems. (Copyright© 2014 Karl Storz and Covidien. All rights reserved. Used with permission of Karl Storz and Covidien.)

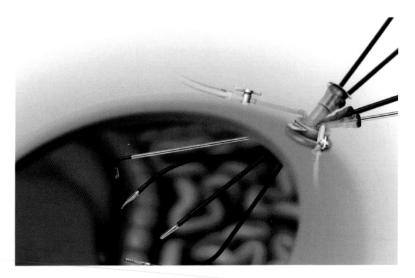

Figure 2. Illustration of a single-port laparoscopic surgery. Note that high-definition laparoscopes with deflectable tips are preferred to provide optimal visualization from any angle. Angulated and articulating laparoscopic instruments are also available to increase the triangulation between the operating hands, although paradoxical movements will be required. (Copyright© 2014 Olympus. All rights reserved. Used with permission of Olympus.)

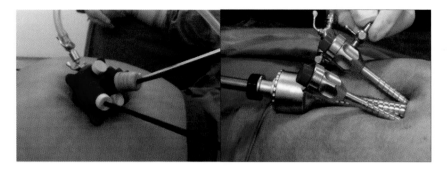

Figure 3. Comparison of a specialized port system on the left, and an improvised single port set-up on the right.

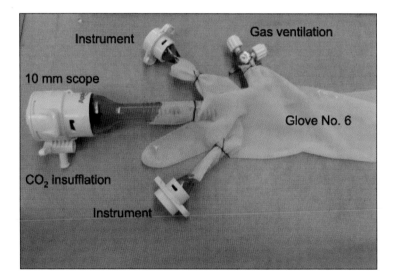

Figure 4. Another example of an improvised single-port system. The fingers of a sterile glove provide the "ports" through which instruments area placed.

opening, with the fingers of the glove left extracorporeally. The laparoscope and instruments are then inserted via the glove's fingers and secured with ties (Fig. 4). These methods are considerably cheaper than the commercially available specialised port systems, though the decision to use one over the other is best guided by individual comfort and preference.

The steps of the operation are no different from the conventional laparoscopic cholecystectomy, besides the larger peri-umbilical incision and the

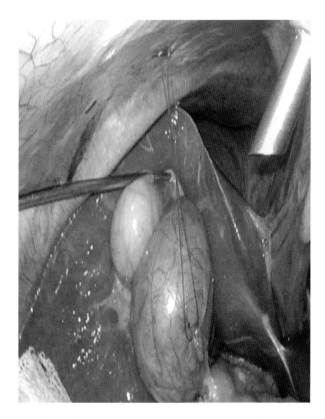

Figure 5. Example of gallbladder suspension with a straight needle. Note that this was done for a laparoscopic cholecystectomy using two subcostal ports only. Incidental finding of a gallbladder duplication.

lack of subcostal ports. As per the two subcostal ports method, the gallbladder is not grasped and lifted over the liver edge due to the absence of subcostal ports.

The lack of gallbladder exposure from upward traction further compounds the difficulty of this approach. One can suspend the gallbladder via a suture passed through the anterior abdominal wall (Fig. 5). Firstly, a straight needle is passed into the peritoneal cavity through the subcostal region, grasped with a forceps and passed through gallbladder fundus or Hartmann's pouch — being careful to pierce only the seromusuclar layer and not into the lumen of the gallbladder. The needle is then passed back through the anterior abdominal wall through a point adjacent to the entry puncture. The gallbladder can now be lifted towards the anterior abdominal wall via manipulation of the suture ends protruding from both the entry and exit sites on the abdominal wall. It is simple and perfectly acceptable to introduce additional ports or needles to aid in dissection or retraction if a pure single incision method proves too challenging.

The crucial difference between single-port laparoscopic cholecystectomy and the conventional laparoscopic cholecystectomy is the loss of triangulation between the two working instruments. Parts of the operation may have to be performed with the instruments crossed over the other in a paradoxical manner, in order to gain that extra critical range of motion. Angulated and articulating laparoscopic instruments have been designed in an attempt to provide increased manoeuvrability and pseudo-triangulation to the surgeon (Fig. 6).

Another challenge to overcome is the frequent conflict between the movement of the laparoscope and the two instruments. Laparoscopes with a flexible lens tip can alleviate some of the congestion, by allowing the laparoscope shaft to be directed away from the surgical field (and the shafts of the working instruments), and yet still be able to visualise the operative field. In addition, laparoscopes with a "chip-on-tip" technology allow for a stream-lined profile with a single coaxial cable and this reduces the issue of clashing with an otherwise bulky camera head (Fig. 7).

Given all the mechanical and ergonomic disadvantages, there is a steep learning curve for single incision laparoscopic cholecystectomy. In carefully selected cases, morbidity and mortality rates are similar when compared to conventional laparoscopic cholecystectomy. Pain score is similar, if not raised, due to the larger peri-umbilical incision and stretching of the rectus sheath by the single-port systems. In addition, there is a slight theoretical increased risk of incisional hernia due to the larger fascia defect, especially with the method that creates multiple fascia defects. The raising of an umbilical flap to accommodate the port systems or extra ports also may lead to increased wound issues like infection or skin necrosis.

Proponents of the single-port method claim superior cosmesis when the incision is done trans-umbilical, and efficacy and safety is similar when done

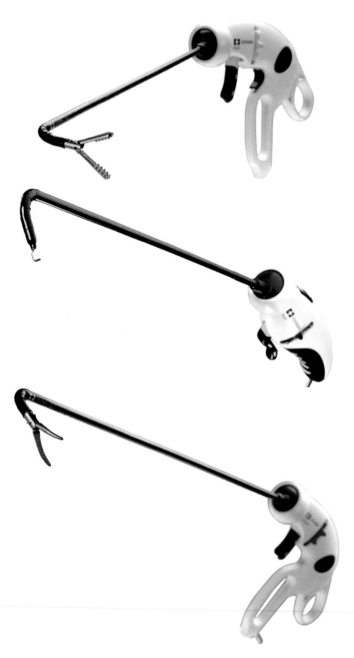

Figure 6.   Examples of articulating instruments used in single incision laparoscopic surgery.
(Copyright© 2014 Covidien. All rights reserved. Used with permission of Covidien.)

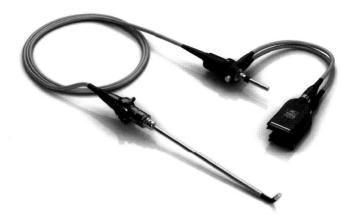

Figure 7. A high-definition laparoscope with "chip-on-tip" technology and coaxial cable commonly used in single incision laparoscopic surgery. (Copyright© 2014 Olympus. All rights reserved. Used with permission of Olympus.)

by experienced surgeons. It is of the authors' opinion that while single-port laparoscopic cholecystectomy has a role to play in uncomplicated cases where patients desire a "scar-less" experience, it cannot be recommended as an equal to the conventional laparoscopic method when dealing with the majority of cases.

Robotic Surgery
for Cholecystectomy

Robotic surgery currently involves the use of the Da Vinci™ system. The system has a remote console where the surgeon sits and operates remotely under non-sterile conditions. The console consists of a 3D screen that projects images captured from the high-definition laparoscope, and hand-held controls that give the surgeon increased freedom of movement and dexterity as compared to laparoscopic surgery. The surgeon also controls the laparoscope's position, which stays fixed to a particular view unless actively moved by the surgeon. Assistants remain in the sterile field and stand beside the patient, assisting in the docking and undocking of the various instruments the surgeon requires in the course of the operation (Fig. 1).

The advantages of robotic surgery include increased dexterity, and the elimination of positional and intention tremors. The 3D images also provide the surgeon with better anatomical definition that is crucial when dealing with delicate structures.

However, robotic surgery is non-tactile, cumbersome, relatively expensive and time-consuming. Each instrument change has to be done manually by an assistant. The camera view while clear and defined is inflexible and alterations in camera views require intermittent pauses in the surgical procedure whilst the surgeon re-adjusts the laparoscope.

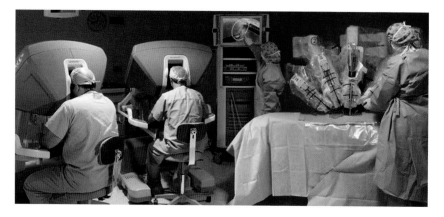

Figure 1. Robotic surgery allows the surgeon to control the instruments remotely from a non-sterilized console. The assistant(s) remain in the sterile field. The assistants' main job will be to insert and remove instruments via different ports as directed by the surgeon. They may also help with retraction using conventional laparoscopic instruments.

Robotic surgery is a relatively new entrant into the world of surgery, but has quickly found a role in a number of operative procedures, ranging from otorhinolaryngology, head and neck surgery, gynaecology, urology and general surgery. The majority of operative procedures that have incorporated robotic surgery into their standard of care have one thing in common: operating in an enclosed and tight anatomical space. This is not true of the surgical field involved in laparoscopic cholecystectomy. Some surgeons combine conventional laparoscopic surgery with robotic surgery to perform different aspects of the procedure; this allows the surgeon to utilise the speed and litheness of conventional laparoscopy for the majority of the operation, while maximising the potential of robotic surgery in enclosed spaces like the pelvic region.

Currently, robotic surgery is not considered the standard of care for cholecystectomy. It may provide some benefit for rare complex cases requiring precision dissection, such as common bile duct exploration or chronic cholecystitis with multiple adhesions, but the increase in cost, peri-operative preparation and operative time is not justified in a routine cholecystectomy.

Until robotic surgery becomes cheaper, more adaptable, and instrument and camera view adjustments become less cumbersome, it will remain largely a novelty for cholecystectomy.

Challenging Scenarios

There is no such thing as a straightforward operation; every procedure undertaken, simple or complex, comes with its own set of potential challenges and complications. The surgical team must always be mindful of this basic tenet, and avoid falling into complacency. There are certain circumstances that need to be recognised as being fraught with more potential landmines than others. These issues can either be pre-existing conditions that are recognised pre-operatively, or events that occur intra-operatively. The scenarios described here are by no means exhaustive, but reflect some of the more commonly encountered difficult ones in practice.

Obese Patient

There are several issues to be considered when treating obese patients. Intubation at the start of the procedure may be more challenging due to the increased amount of soft tissue around the oropharyngeal area. The use of special instruments such as fibre-optic laryngoscopes may aid the anaesthetist greatly.

Lung compliance is decreased in obese patients due to a thicker chest wall and increased abdominal wall tension, making ventilation during surgery more difficult. This is further exacerbated by the pneumoperitoneum created during surgery.

Such patients are more likely to have other comorbidities comprising the metabolic syndrome. These include hypertension, hyperlipidaemia and diabetes mellitus. End organ damage is not uncommon as well, and includes ischaemic heart disease, prior cerebrovascular accidents, peripheral vascular disease and renal impairment. These conditions increase the risk involved in anaesthesia and surgery, thereby warranting more care during the peri-operative period for such individuals.

Technically, the body frame and intra-abdominal anatomy of obese patients may also pose challenges to the surgeon. A thicker abdominal wall may necessitate the need for longer laparoscopic ports. Additionally, it also hinders the pivoting movements of instruments. Gaining access to the peritoneum via the open Hassan method through the thick abdominal wall is similarly challenging. However, using the method described in the prior chapters is usually foolproof, with only extra time needed to traverse the thick adipose layer. Otherwise, one may elect to use an optical trocar-port system if available.

Increased pressures will also be needed in creating a pneumoperitoneum with sufficient working space required for surgery. This potentially decreases venous return to the point of cardiac decompensation. Large, thick omentum and bulky mesenteric fat are common in obese patients, and constrains optimal visualisation during surgery. It is also not uncommon for these patients to have a fatty, bulky liver with a lower edge that can flop over the gallbladder and obscure access. The use of gauze strips in such cases to retract mesentery, bowel, liver and omentum to create adequate operative space becomes invaluable in such patients (Fig. 1).

Liver Cirrhosis

Liver dysfunction as a result of cirrhosis leads to physiological impairments and anatomical anomalies that can complicate the peri-operative period and increase risk of surgical complications (Fig. 2).

Deficiencies of the coagulation pathway and thrombocytopenia from hypersplenism can cause increased blood loss intra-operatively. It is also a risk factor for post-operative haemorrhage from the surgical bed and incision sites. Patients may require the transfusion of blood products pre-operatively and intra-operatively to correct these disorders of the clotting pathway.

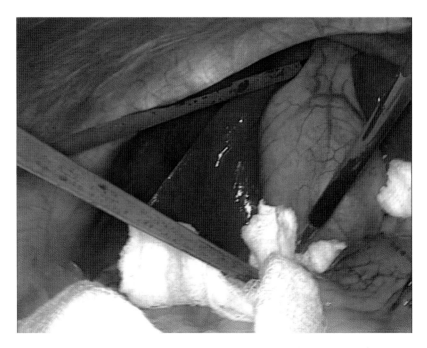

Figure 1. Multiple gauze strips may be needed to pack away omentum, mesentery, and a capacious stomach in obese patients.

Patients with ascites may face the issue of limited working space even with peritoneal insufflation, and possible cardiac decompensation from high intra-abdominal pressures. It is not uncommon for umbilical hernias to develop as a result of long-standing ascites; this further complicates periumbilical port placement. If small, the umbilical hernia can be repaired with simple interrupted sutures after an incision has been made through the umbilical skin, making sure to catch the fascia securely. Larger hernias may necessitate the use of a prosthetic mesh for repair.

In the presence of portal hypertension and a canalised falciform ligament, a supraumbilical port placement is contraindicated. In severe cases, the collateral circulation around the umbilicus may rule out periumbilical port placement entirely. The working instrument port that is placed just right of the falciform ligament can potentially cause massive bleeding if it lacerates the re-canalised vessel within the falciform ligament. Portal hypertension can also cause the development of engorged collateral vessels around

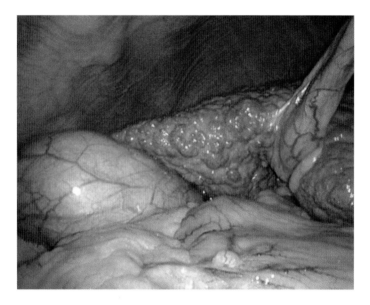

Figure 2.   Intra-operative image from patient with liver cirrhosis. Note the knobbly surface of the liver.

the hepatobiliary tree and gallbladder bed, from branches of the hepatic, left gastric and gastroduodenal arteries. All these increase the risk of haemorrhage.

Post-operatively, wound healing in patients with liver cirrhosis may be affected due to nutritional deficiencies in proteins and amino acids. Patients are also at increased risk of wound breakdown and infection. Uncommonly, the stress from surgery and ensuing catabolic state may precipitate hepatic encephalopathy.

Bile Spillage

Spillage of bile intra-operatively, though not strictly a complication, is an undesired occurrence and may lead to complications if corrective measures are not taken intra-operatively. Bile is considered to be infected in approximately 30% of cholecystectomies and its spillage within the abdominal cavity poses a risk of a post-operative infected intra-abdominal collection.

Bile spillage is more common in inflammatory conditions, when the oedema and/or fibrosis obliterate the normally avascular tissue plane between the gallbladder and the liver. When the gallbladder is inadvertently entered, the surgeon should attempt to grasp the gallbladder at the point of perforation to limit the spillage. If this manoeuvre can prevent continuous leakage, then it is tolerable for the operation to proceed. However, some gallbladders will require evacuation of bile via the perforation with the suction apparatus to avert widespread contamination. Some oedematous pyogenic gallbladders actually benefit from such decompression, allowing them to be grasped much easier.

Gauze strips routinely placed around the gallbladder help limit the area of contamination, and in most cases, do a satisfactory job of containing spilled gallstones (Figs. 3 and 4). In the absence of gauze strips during profuse leakage, the bile can potentially track to the subphrenic, subhepatic and right pericolic spaces. There is controversy regarding whether meticulous suctioning or irrigation with suction is the best approach in dealing with peritoneal contamination. In our practice, we feel that copious irrigation allows for dilution of contaminants and more comprehensive clearing of debris.

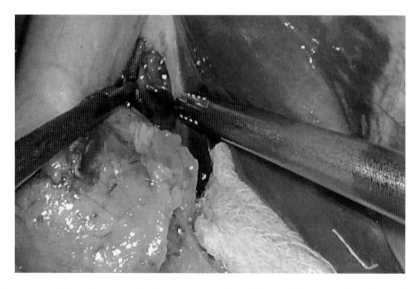

Figure 3. Bile spillage after inadvertent perforation of the gallbladder can be mitigated by suction and copious irrigation. The presence of gauze around the site of leakage helps to control the peritoneal contamination.

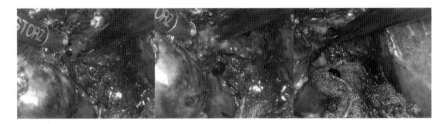

Figure 4. Suctioning and irrigation can mitigate accidental bile spillage. Gauze strips are useful for limiting the contamination of the peritoneal cavity, and also to trap gallstones.

Where peritoneal contamination is extensive, drains can be placed in the dependent subhepatic or subphrenic spaces even if no remnant contamination is visualised. As the patient is usually supine during the operation, some residual contamination may not be readily visible. Repositioning of the patient with a slight reverse Tredenlenburg manoeuvre may be helpful in allowing contaminated fluid in the subphrenic space to gravitate caudally.

Porcelain Gallbladder

Porcelain gallbladder arises from dystrophic calcification of the gallbladder wall as a result of chronic inflammation, most commonly secondary to gallstones. It is an absolute indication for surgery even in the absence of symptoms, due to its increased risk of harbouring or developing gallbladder carcinoma.

The gallbladder may be adhered to adjacent organs due to the inflammatory process, making visualisation more challenging. Its hard, glass-like wall may preclude grasping it with forceps; a large bowel forceps with its jaws held open can be utilised to suspend the gallbladder from its base, in a scooping action. Perforation of the gallbladder should be avoided, due to possible peritoneal seeding of cancer cells if indeed the gallbladder is harbouring an occult or early carcinoma.

Pre-operative diagnostic work-up is especially important in patients recognised to have porcelain gallbladder, and further radiological or endoscopic investigations should be performed to assess the likelihood of carcinoma (Fig. 5). These may include MRCP or endoscopic ultrasound (EUS). Prior to proceeding with laparoscopic cholecystectomy, the surgeon should perform a full diagnostic laparoscopic examination, focusing on the

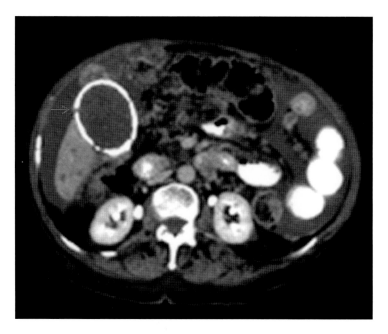

Figure 5. Axial section of a computer tomography showing a porcelain gallbladder with its calcified wall (red arrow).

hepatobiliary area to look for indications of malignancy. These include enlarged lymph nodes, peritoneal deposits and gross invasion of the gallbladder into adjacent structures. Laparoscopic ultrasound (LUS) may be of use, although not routinely performed.

If there does not appear to be any suggestion of malignancy based on pre-operative evaluation, the operation is carried out in the routine manner with care not to cause gallbladder perforation (Fig. 6). Tumours advanced enough to cause local invasion, lymphatic, hepatic, or peritoneal spread should be picked up on pre-operative imaging. In the unfortunate event that an inadequate diagnostic work-up was performed and there is gross evidence of tumour intra-operatively, the operation is best abandoned and the patient re-counselled on the need for either a radical cholecystectomy with liver resection (if invading through the submucosa but deemed to be curable), palliative surgery (if widespread local, lymphatic or peritoneal spread) for symptoms and possible biliary obstruction, or the role of chemotherapy.

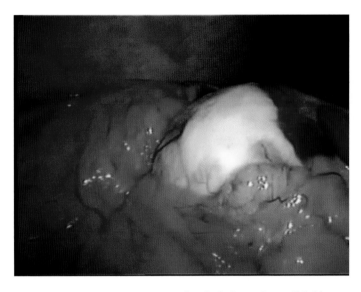

Figure 6. Intra-operative view of a calcified porcelain gallbladder.

The non-pliable nature of the gallbladder may require its piecemeal removal via the umbilicus. This may provide a technical challenge for the pathologist, especially with regards to submucosal invasion by a potential carcinoma. Even with piecemeal removal, the periumbilical incision usually needs to be widened, which increases the risk of incisional hernia formation.

Empyema and Gangrenous Cholecystitis

The severe inflammatory nature of empyema and gangrenous cholecystitis increases the likelihood of extensive adhesions, and bleeding is more likely to occur during dissection. Finding the correct plane to dissect the gallbladder from its surrounding tissue may be challenging. Gallbladder perforation and spillage are more common in such cases (see above).

In cases where the gallbladder is engorged to the point where grasping it becomes an issue, the surgeon can elect to decompress the gallbladder to avoid unintentional perforation (Figs. 7 and 8). This can be carried out with a laparoscopic needle decompressor, usually through the port below the

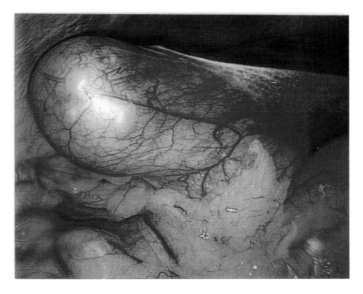

Figure 7. A grossly distended gallbladder filled with pus.

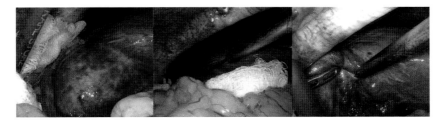

Figure 8. The empyematous gallbladder appears swollen and necrotic. Using a laparoscopic needle aspirator, the gallbladder can be emptied of its contents, making it easier it be grasped and manipulated.

xiphoid process (Figs. 9 and 10). If the needle fails to penetrate the chronically thickened wall, a deliberate small perforation can be made in the gallbladder with hook diathermy, and the decompression subsequently performed by the suction apparatus via the hole made.

The relevant anatomical landmarks such as Calot's triangle, Cloquet's node and the cystic artery, may not be readily appreciable due to oedema and iatrogenic haemorrhage caused by dissection. Here, the use of gauze

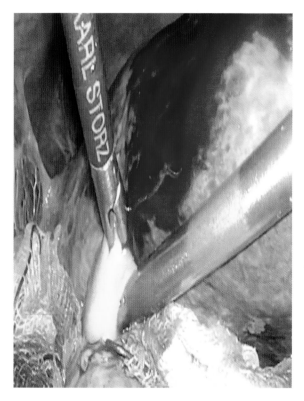

Figure 9.   Gross pus leakage in an empyematous gallbladder.

strips helps greatly in the exposure and dissection of vital structures. A gauze strip held with a forceps is a great blunt dissecting tool. In addition, it soaks up blood and oil to maintain a relatively dry operative field. It also provides a white background to enhance the colour contrast of the patient's anatomy to allow the surgeon to better identify structures. Placing gauze strips around the area of dissection can alert the surgeon to the accidental injury of biliary structures, when the leaking bile stains the white gauze.

To avoid the catastrophic complication of common bile duct injury during particularly difficult cholecystectomies, some surgeons recommend a subtotal cholecystectomy, in which the portion of the gallbladder including the neck and the cystic duct is left *in situ* and untouched. This purportedly

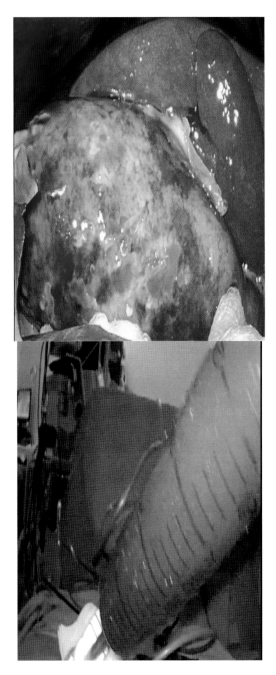

Figure 10. Severe gangrenous cholecystitis. To facilitate grasping and dissection of the gallbladder, the gallbladder was decompressed with thick infected bile aspirated.

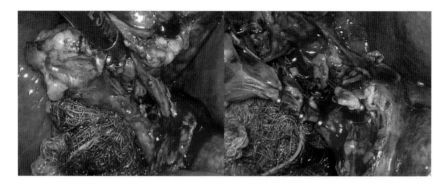

Figure 11.   Identification of Calot's triangle, whilst difficult, can be achieved with patience even in a severe acutely inflamed gallbladder.

leaves the Calot's triangle untouched with lesser risk of biliary injury. However, we believe this to be a suboptimal approach, as the remnant gallbladder is still prone to future inflammation, especially if a gallstone is lodged in the cystic duct or gallbladder neck.

While the cystic duct may be the location of a lodged stone causing cholecystitis, it is almost never involved in the inflammatory process itself. With meticulous and careful dissection using a variety of techniques such as blunt and sharp dissection, cautery, and irrigation, the cystic duct can almost always be identified and secured (Figs. 11 and 12).

Multiple Adhesions

Adhesions can occur as a consequence of the inflammatory process involving the gallbladder; in such cases it is limited to the gallbladder, omentum, duodenum, liver, and rarely, the colon in the right upper quadrant. A combination of sharp dissection with scissors, cautery using forceps or a hook, or blunt dissection with gauze and forceps can help with adhesiolysis (Fig. 13). It is essential to create enough working space for the surgeon to visualise the structures to ensure patient safety. Diathermy is not advisable when taking down adhesions close to bowel; sharp dissection with scissors offers better control and is preferred. Diathermy is useful in haemostasis during dissection especially when dealing with omental adhesions.

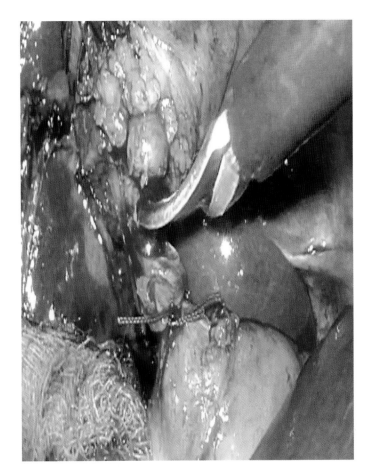

Figure 12. If the cystic duct does prove to be too thick for the application of clips, sutures can be used to secure the cystic duct as well.

Adhesions are commonly encountered as an outcome of previous surgeries performed in the right and left upper quadrants, or from midline incisions. Adhesions in the right upper quadrant can be dealt with similarly to adhesions secondary to gallbladder inflammation (Fig. 14). These tend to be more adhesive, but less vascular due to their chronicity. Acute adhesions due to an on-going inflammatory process, however, can be trickier to deal with due to their increased oedema and vascularity (Figs. 15 and 16).

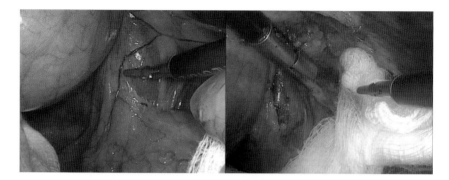

Figure 13.   Adhesions can be tackled with diathermy, or with blunt dissection. Laparoscopic scissors can also be utilised.

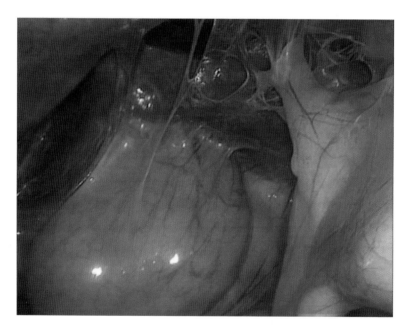

Figure 14.   Multiple chronic adhesions affecting the right hypochondrium, involving the liver, gallbladder, colon and stomach (not shown).

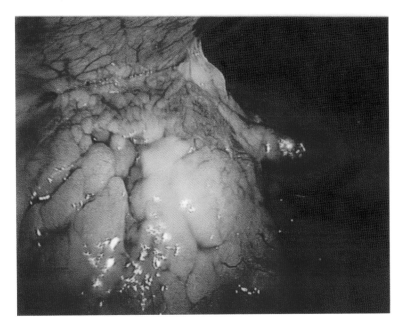

Figure 15. Acute omental adhesions engulfing the gallbladder in a severe case of gallbladder empyema.

Of particular concern are adhesions that are centred on the umbilicus due to previous midline incisions. These can obstruct the initial Hassan cannulation, and cause haemorrhage. Particularly, a loop of small bowel may be adhered to or around the point of entry of the Hassan cannula and thus be injured during peritoneal entry. It is essential for the surgeon to inspect the small bowel loops after pneumoperitoneum has been achieved to recognise potential small bowel injury and take remedial actions. A 5 mm laparoscope may have to be inserted from one of the working ports to enable full visualisation of any adhesions to the umbilical area. In situations where Hassan cannulation is hindered by adhesions at the periumbilical area, an alternative method would be to enter the peritoneum via a different site. Alternatively, creation of the pneumoperitoneum by the Veress needle method away from sites of potential adhesions may be considered.

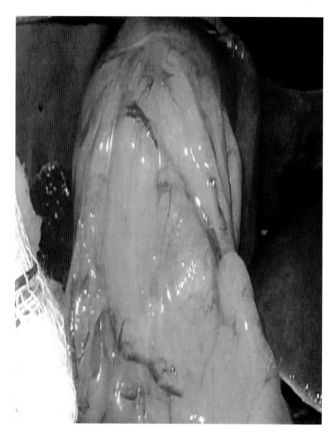

Figure 16.   Omental adhesions over the gallbladder in a case of acute chlecystitis.

Cholecysto-enteric Fistulas

This is a rare condition stemming from the on-going inflammation chronic cholecystitis coupled with unfortunate anatomical proximity of the adjacent small or large bowel. As the inflammatory process progresses, an abnormal fistulous track develops between the gallbladder and the involved segment of bowel (Fig. 17).

If the duodenum is involved, it is usually at its second portion. The duodenum is initially adherent to the gallbladder, but over time repeat episodes of inflammation and fibrosis causes an abnormal track to form between the gallbladder fundus and the duodenum. This condition is far more common in the elderly due to the time period it takes for the fistula to

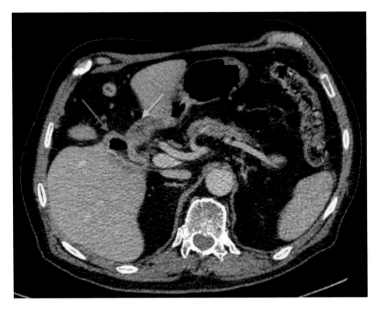

Figure 17. A case of cholecystoduodenal fistula. The gallbladder with air within (green arrow) is seen adherent to a collapsed duodenum (yellow arrow).

form, and its usual presentation is actually small bowel obstruction due to passed gallstones obstructing the ileocaecal valve.

The large bowel can also be involved, resulting in what is known as a cholecysto-colonic fistula, which usually is limited to the length of bowel from the hepatic flexure to the proximal transverse colon.

Strictly speaking, cholecystectomy may not be necessary if the presenting complaint is small bowel obstruction. This is because the fistula frequently attains drainage of the gallbladder. Indeed all that is usually needed would be an enterotomy with removal of the offending gallstone followed by primary repair. If there are remnant gallstones in the gallbladder, which may potentially cause a recurrence of gallstone-induced small bowel obstruction, or evidence of on-going cholecystitis, then cholecystectomy is indicated. This should be performed in the same setting as the small bowel enterotomy, and can be completed laparoscopically.

The surgery will be technically more demanding due to the presence of adhesions, isolation of the fistula track and the need for the duodenal wall defect to be sutured securely. However, results are excellent if the tract can be well delineated, and the enteric defect sutured securely intracorporeally.

Frequently Asked Questions

An operation, no matter how seemingly straightforward, should never be taken lightly. It is normal for patients to have questions regarding the operation, risks and its outcomes. Often, these concerns are common among patients. We will attempt to deal with the more frequently queried topics here.

Particularly, we will focus on the post-operative experience of patients and deal with the impact a laparoscopic cholecystectomy has on a patient's life.

(1) How long will I have to stay in hospital following a laparoscopic cholecystectomy?

Patients who have an uneventful operation can expect a speedy discharge. Most are discharged within 24 hours, with more complicated cases staying for 2–3 days. Your surgical team will monitor your progress and update you on the expected duration of post-operative hospital stay after the operation.

(2) How long does recovery take following a laparoscopic cholecystectomy?

The actual length of recovery will depend on a number of factors. These include pre-existing co-morbidities, nature of surgery and patient's post-operative lifestyle.

Pre-existing Co-morbidities

Patients without any pre-existing medical conditions such as cardiovascular, renal, hepatic, gastrointestinal and/or oncological disease may expect to make a quick recovery ranging from a few days to a week following surgery. Patients with existing co-morbidities may or may not experience complications but may be required to spend a day or two longer in hospital for observation and may expect to make a recovery from the laparoscopic cholecystectomy by about two weeks post surgery typically, depending on the severity of the pre-existing condition.

Nature of Surgery

Recovery from a laparoscopic cholecystectomy is typically quicker than that of open cholecystectomy provided the laparoscopic procedure has been carried out competently, and that patients do not experience any surgical complications. By virtue of the smaller incisions made in a laparoscopic cholecystectomy, post-operative pain is usually less, and wound healing is faster. Laparoscopic cholecystectomy typically involves up to four small incisions no bigger than 10 mm being made in various positions on the abdomen. Through these small "keyholes", surgical instruments are introduced into the body and the procedure carried out. Compared to open cholecystectomy, which involves a single incision roughly 10–12 cm in length, the aesthetic and surgical benefits of laparoscopic cholecystectomy clearly outweigh those of open cholecystectomy. Patients are typically discharged after staying one day at the hospital and have their stitches removed 5–7 days after the procedure if required.

Post-operative Lifestyle

Patients are usually advised to avoid strenuous activities for roughly a week after the procedure. They are also encouraged to adopt a simple and "soft" diet during this period and are recommended to increase their intake of fluids. The return to normal dietary habits should be carried out gradually and judiciously, and foods that are high in fat content should be kept to a minimum during the recovery period.

(3) What are some of the symptoms I can expect post-operatively?

The most common symptom patients will have is wound pain, which is usually worst at the wound around the belly-button or umbilicus. In cases of gallbladder inflammation, there may be pain around the right upper part of the abdomen, which is due to the inflammation of the abdominal lining in that area. These can usually be controlled adequately with pain-killers.

Some patients will experience some degree of nausea and vomiting, which is a common side effect of the general anaesthesia given during the operation. This will usually be resolved by the next day, and patients should be encouraged to take as much fluids as they can manage orally. Medications to prevent nausea and vomiting commonly help alleviate these symptoms.

(4) What are some of the risks and common complications?

Removal of the gallbladder is one of the most common operations performed today, and is usually a safe procedure. However, there are some well-recognised complications that may arise.

Bleeding can occur during the operation from blood vessels near the liver, or the liver itself. This is usually easily managed, but may require a conversion to the open method of surgery if it cannot be controlled. Very infrequently, bleeding can arise following the operation, and may compel the need for further intervention.

Injury of the organs near the gallbladder occasionally occurs, and may require repair during the operation, with or without a conversion to the open method of surgery. The repair itself may be simple or necessitate a major operation depending on the nature and severity of the organ injury. Commonly injured structures include the bile ducts, liver, stomach, small intestines and large intestines. There are rare cases where the injury is not noticed during the initial operation, and only detected up later. Depending on the nature and severity of the injury, further procedures or operations may be necessary to rectify the situation.

Wound infections are uncommon in an otherwise uncomplicated gallbladder removal operation. It usually manifests around 4–5 days after the operation, and can be suspected when there is increased redness, swelling or tenderness around the wound(s). Most are superficial, and will resolve with a course of antibiotics. More challenging cases may require the opening of the superficial part of the wound to allow drainage of the infection. If severe, wound infections can increase one's risk of subsequent scar and hernia formation.

Some groups of patients may be more at risk than others for certain complications, based on their gallbladder condition or other medical conditions. Patients are advised to speak to their surgeon regarding their individual risk for the common complications that may arise.

(5) How will the removal of the gallbladder affect my life?

This is a usual concern that most patients have. Many are worried about how a missing gallbladder will affect their overall health and lifestyle. As discussed in earlier chapters, there is minimal impact. The gallbladder stores excess bile produced by the liver and serves as a reservoir of bile. After a meal, the gallbladder contracts and expels its bilious contents into the common bile duct via the cystic duct. The bile then flows into the duodenum where it aids in the emulsification of fats and increases the efficiency of fat digestion. The gallbladder thus serves no function other than storage and concentration of excess bile, and does not itself produce bile. Even without the gallbladder, bile is continuously synthesised in the liver and secreted into the common bile duct.

(6) Does this mean that the amount of bile released into the small intestine after a meal will drop?

Yes. The gallbladder usually serves as a reservoir of bile that is used after ingestion of food. This, in addition to the constant baseline flow of bile secreted by the liver, translates into a larger volume of bile involved in digestion. With the removal of the gallbladder, the patient will have a reduced volume of bile released after meals. Thus, the only impact of a missing gallbladder would be a diminished volume of bile involved in digestion, with a consequent lowered rate of fat digestion following a meal.

(7) Are there any types of food I should avoid after the removal of the gallbladder?

The removal of the gallbladder should not interfere greatly with your usual diet and there are generally no strict restrictions on the types of food or drink you are allowed to consume post-operatively. However, it is recommended that in the weeks following the removal of the gallbladder, food high in fat content should not be consumed in large quantities, as your digestive system may not be able to cope. In due time, the rate of bile secretion may be increased as your body adjusts to life without a gallbladder, but the rate at which your digestive system processes fat may never reach pre-operative levels.

(8) Will my bowel habits be affected or changed?

In the initial few months after the gall bladder has been removed, you may notice an increase in the frequency of having to empty your bowels especially after a meal high in fat content. The stools may be oily or float on the surface due to the relatively high composition of undigested fat.

(9) How long will this take before my bowel patterns return to normal?

Every patient is unique in terms of health and lifestyle. There is no fixed time frame that applies to all. Factors such as diet, health status, physical activity and overall lifestyle play a part. By understanding the relationship between what they eat and their bowel patterns, patients are in the best position to manage such changes. Most patients are able to adjust their dietary intake satisfactorily and report no decrease in their quality of life.

With time, your digestive system should be able to cope with the digestion of normal fat intake. However, excessive intake of foods high in fats and cholesterol should generally be avoided as part of a healthy lifestyle and moderation in eating habits.

(10) Are there medications I can take to get rid of gallstones instead of having surgery to remove the gallbladder? What about traditional Chinese medicine or other traditional herbal remedies?

Pharmaceutical agents currently available on the market to eliminate gallstones contain bile acids as the principal ingredient, and work by altering the concentration of the various components of bile in order to promote the dissolution of gallstones. However, patients have to be on the drug for a significant period stretching up to 18 months before appreciating any noticeable benefits. Moreover, the efficacy of such therapeutic agents is restricted in terms of the type of gallstones they are able to dissolve. Small gallstones with high cholesterol content generally respond to these drugs while pigmented, calcified stones larger than 15 mm in diameter do not. The cost of oral dissolution therapy is also higher in the long term, and patients have to remain on the drug for the foreseeable future, as ceasing drug therapy will result in the return of gallstones. There is also a significant probability of gallstone recurrences even while a patient is on oral dissolution therapy. As a consequence, oral therapeutics are only moderately effective and do not appear promising in terms of managing gallstones or providing a satisfactory resolution to individuals suffering from chronic cholecystitis. They are usually offered as an option to patients who have gallstones which may respond, and/or who are poor surgical candidates.

With regards to traditional medicine, there is insufficient empirical research and evidence to support the safety and efficacy of traditional therapies. Some traditional drugs and herbs may also contain chemical compounds that may interact with conventional medications with adverse effects. Patients should therefore be judicious in their use of such alternative therapies and consult with their doctor before attempting traditional remedies.

(11) Is there a chance of my gallbladder being cancerous?

Gallbladder cancers, if suspected before the operation, should not be attempted to be removed via the key-hole or laparoscopic method. These cases usually require a more complicated surgery via the open method.

Certain gallbladder conditions increase the risk of gallbladder cancer, including calcium deposition in the gallbladder and chronic gallbladder inflammation. In the absence of such conditions, the risk of gallbladder cancer is exceedingly low.

There are rare cases, where a gallbladder cancer is identified after the operation when the removed gallbladder is sent for routine microscopic examination. Further treatment, including surgery or chemotherapy may be required, and is best discussed on an individualised basis with the surgeon.

Conclusion

The use of laparoscopy ushered in a new age for surgery. Cholecystectomy has come a long way, from the days of an operation with high morbidity and a large scar, to the almost scar-less procedure that can even be performed as day surgery. With rising affluence of the population, symptomatic gallstone disease can be expected to rise in the future. The increasing sophistication of patients, coupled with a generation of young surgeons accustomed to the minimally invasive approach, will drive the demand for innovations that will allow for further minimally invasive methods.

The development of more precise 3D systems, more advanced instrumentation and hand-held robotic systems will no doubt be forthcoming. Such progress will further enhance the safety of laparoscopic surgery and translate into better outcomes for our patients. As we surge into the age of robotics and nanotechnology, it is not far-fetched to imagine that one day not too long in the future, fully independent robots may be able to perform operations in a minimally invasive manner.

Will the relevance of surgeons be threatened by the exponential growth in complexities and intricacies of robotic systems? Whichever way forward, patient safety and good surgical outcomes must always be of paramount importance before any new technology is embraced. As custodians of the patients' well-being, surgeons must be equipped with the skills to provide competent surgical care, and take a life-long approach to learning and mastering new surgical techniques as they develop.

Appendix:
Equipment

Manufacturers are constantly looking to push the frontiers when it comes to surgical instruments, and those used in the field of laparoscopy have seen significant advances since its inception in the 1980s. Current laparoscopic equipment has evolved from rudimentary beginnings to the precision tools of today, and they will only get better with further technological innovations.

Whilst knowledge of the finer technical details of the many electrical components of surgical equipment in the operating room are not required for their proper application, and are best left to the manufacturers and engineers, surgeons and operating room staff do require a working understanding of the equipment they are handling. This will allow them to optimise the potential of the equipment at their disposal, take the necessary safety precautions, as well as perform basic troubleshooting when the need arises.

Endoscopic Camera System

A laparoscope is a fibre-optic camera mounted on the tip of a shaft, with a light source providing illumination attached to the base of the shaft. The laparoscope used is usually 5 mm or 10 mm in diameter, and has a viewing angle of typically 0° or 30°, though different angulations are also available. The 30° camera is most commonly used for laparoscopic cholecystectomy. An angled camera allows for shifting of the visual field to the left or right when the attachment of the light cable at the base of the laparoscope shaft is

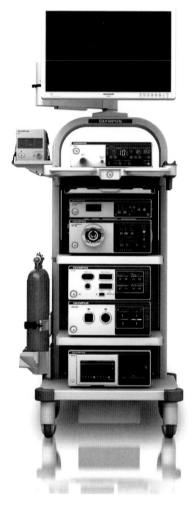

Figure 1.   The laparoscopy tower, for economy of space and ease of movement, is an essential equipment for laparoscopic surgery. From top to bottom, the components of the equipment are: high-definition monitor, gas-insufflator (gas canister is located at bottom left of the trolley), video system centre, light source, two types of energy sources, DVD recorder. (Copyright© 2014 Olympus. All rights reserved. Used with permission of Olympus.)

rotated to the right or left respectively. This allows for more flexibility in achieving suitable views during surgery (Figs. 2 and 3). Newer laparoscopes now come with deflectable tips that allow for a 360° view of the surgical field from a stationary position; tip movement in the up-down and left-right direction are controlled by different dials at the base of the laparoscope (Fig. 4).

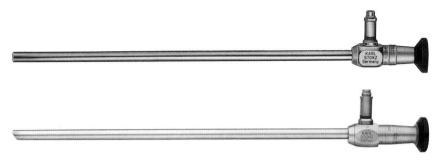

Figure 2. Standard laparoscopes. The top example is a 0° laparoscope, while the bottom example is a 30° laparoscope. (Copyright© 2014 Karl Storz. All rights reserved. Used with permission of Karl Storz.)

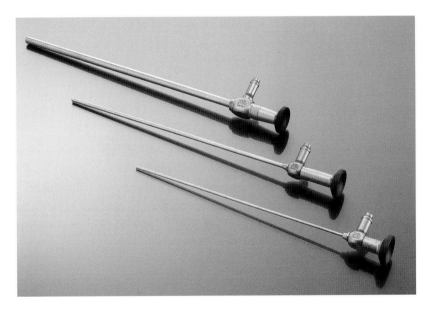

Figure 3. Laparoscopes of different sizes. From top to bottom, 10 mm, 5 mm, 3 mm. (Copyright© 2014 Karl Storz. All rights reserved. Used with permission of Karl Storz.)

The telescope captures images via a distal-mounted objective lens, which are then routed through a rod-lens system to a proximal-mounted ocular lens that magnifies it for the surgeon. Generally, larger telescopes with lower magnification produce images with higher resolution. However, there is a limit to how wide the lens of a telescope can be made before the benefits of minimally invasive surgery are lost. Modern high-definition (HD) endoscopes allow for a noticeably better imaging even with small endoscopes

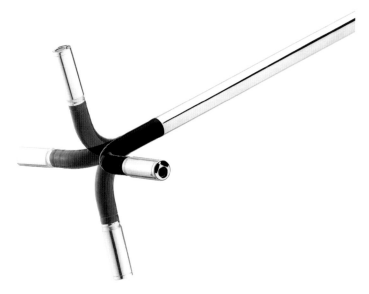

Figure 4.   A HD laparoscope with a deflectable tip. Dials on the camera head control the tip motion. (Copyright© 2014 Olympus. All rights reserved. Used with permission of Olympus.)

displaying a full-circle image on a monitor. Lens design and production quality are also critical factors in determining resolution.

A light source is essential in endoscopic imaging, and the quality of images produced by HD cameras depends very much on high-performance light sources. The illumination provided must possess true-colour properties, brilliant image presentation, sufficient brightness and contrast, and adequate operative field exposure.

Newer, LED light sources are environmentally friendly, and have been found to be economically effective when used in conjunction with HD cameras. Some light sources boast of a safety feature that adopts the "standby" mode when the light source cable detaches from the scope, decreasing the risk of thermal and retinal injury to patients and staff by the light source. Because HD cameras have lower sensitivity due to smaller pixel size, a powerful 300W Xenon light source is often used.

The main difference between standard definition (SD) and HD video formats is best explained by comparing the vertical and horizontal resolutions. Typical SD formats offer a 4:3 aspect ratio, 640 by 480 horizontal and vertical lines; while the HD format provides a 16:9 aspect ratio, 1280 by 720 horizontal and vertical lines. The 1080 HD standard also offers a 16:9 aspect ratio, but 1920 by 1080 horizontal and vertical lines. The temporal resolution is the quantity of captured images expressed as frames per second (fps). The 720p standard represents progressive scanning, capturing the whole frame as you image 60 times per second. The 1080i standard represents interlaced scanning-capturing two fields of half images with alternating lines that are then combined to produce each complete frame. Progressive scanning offers twice the temporal resolution when compared to interlaced scanning, allowing it to capture both fast-moving objects and still images. This allows a quasi-3D image to be formed that may make anatomical structures more visible.

The fitting over images captured by a circular telescope onto a rectangular monitor screen is accomplished by over framing the look, which allows the monitor screen to be completely filled with the surgical image. Wide-screen image acquisition increases the horizontal field of view and decreases the vertical field of view, and is advantageous when the laparoscopic instruments enter the field of view laterally. Withdrawing the laparoscope allows for a panoramic view and makes amends for the loss of vertical field of view.

The camera head consists of a goal lens, a prism assembly and three sensors for acquiring the primary colours of the image. Some camera heads incorporate an optical zoom for adjusting the magnification. Three-chip cameras are currently the accepted standard due to their more natural colour reproduction (Fig. 5).

The camera central computing unit (CCU) connects various aspects of the HD imaging chain, capturing and processing video signals from the camera head for display on the monitor, as well as for transfer to existing recording and printing devices. In addition to processing digital HD images, the CCU should be able to either down-convert HD signals to SD or up-convert SD signals to HD. This will allow the synchrony of different units purchased over a period of technological advancement without resulting in an unacceptable number of obsolete units. In a typical operating room setting, a mixture of SD and HD imaging components is likely to be found. The CCU should be able to accommodate both SD and HD input and, conversely, it will have two digital video outputs — digital video interface (DVI) for the HD signal, and serial digital interface (SDI) for the SD signal.

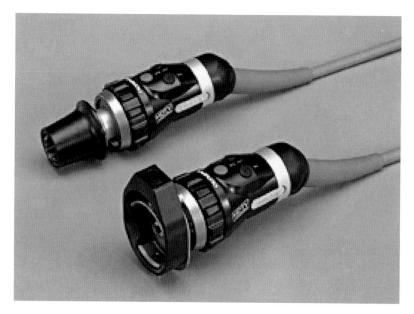

Figure 5. Examples of commercially available camera heads. The top example is a "quick lock" type head, while the bottom example is an "eye piece" type head. There are various models of camera heads on the market, each having their own method of operation. It is important for camera assistants to be familiar with the camera head he/she is operating. (Copyright© 2014 Olympus. All rights reserved. Used with permission of Olympus.)

Video cables that carry digital image data between the camera head, camera CCU, and monitoring and recording devices must offer sufficient bandwidth for video transmission of HD data over long distances. Using the introduction of optical fibre, DVI cabling can now achieve this purpose, and represents the simplest way of transmitting a signal (Fig. 6).

A 26" HD monitor provides clear, brilliant images on a spacious, wide-screen display. It offers both 4:3 and 16:9 aspect ratio display formats, improved colour reproduction and new picture-by-picture capabilities. A monitor displaying images acquired in 16:9 formats enables surgeons to experience more natural vision, and visualisation is much more in tune with human anatomy. For surgeons, this wider, natural view is less straining on the eyes during procedures (Fig. 1).

To achieve the full benefit of HD imaging and maximise performance, the monitor resolution must be properly matched to the camera head acquisition resolution. This may require the de-interlacing, or up-converting of signals to complement the monitor format.

Laparoscope warmers are used occasionally to decrease the temperature differential between the laparoscope tip and the abdominal cavity; laparoscopes are placed within the warmer in a sterile manner approximately 10–15 minutes prior to the surgery. This attempts to mitigate the fogging phenomenon observed on laparoscope tips when inserted into the abdomen — a source of much frustration for many a surgeon. Anti-fog solutions are also available, which are dripped unto a sponge, after which they are gently applied onto the laparoscope tip. Their mechanism is by way of minimising surface tension, resulting in a non-scattering film of water instead of single droplets, an effect called "wetting" (Fig. 7).

Some recent commercial products allow for intra-operative warming of laparoscope tip in an attempt to decrease fogging. They are usually battery-operated, and can fit laparoscopes of different sizes with the use of an adaptor (Fig. 8).

Another method that has been used to prevent fogging intra-operatively is the active removal of plume from electrocautery away from the peritoneal cavity. This is especially important in challenging cases, where the plume from blood and fat being cauterised can severely hamper the surgical team's

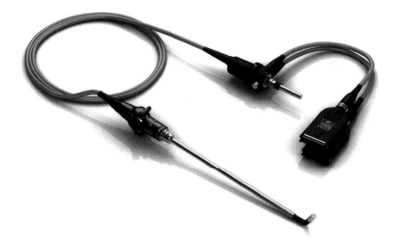

Figure 6. A HD laparoscopic camera system. The light source connector is the short-pointed rod at the proximal end of the device. The video cable carries the image signals back to the CCU via its proximal connecting end. (Copyright© 2014 Olympus. All rights reserved. Used with permission of Olympus.)

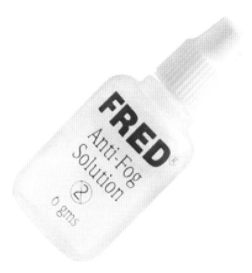

Figure 7.   FRED™, an example of an anti-fog solution commonly used. (Copyright© 2014 Covidien. All rights reserved. Used with permission of Covidien.)

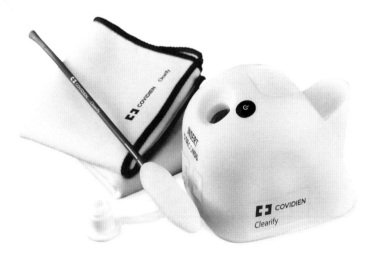

Figure 8.   A commercially available laparoscope warmer system, Clearify™ is shown above. The tip of the laparoscope is inserted into the dock, which has a battery-operated warmer located within. Sponge-tips of two different sizes mounted on opposite ends of a stick allows for cleaning of laparoscopic ports. A cloth is also provided for non-abrasive cleaning of the laparoscope tip. In addition, an adaptor is attached which allows a smaller sized laparoscope to be inserted into the dock. (Copyright© 2014 Covidien. All rights reserved. Used with permission of Covidien.)

view. This can be done manually by the surgeon using a suction device (see below), or passively by releasing a lever on one of the ports that will allow plume to passively escape. However, these usually result in a decrease in the intra-abdominal gas pressure, which can also hinder the surgical view and operative space. A third option is to employ an automated suction-insufflator device that pumps gas into the peritoneal cavity at the same rate it removes it, thereby maintaining a near-constant intra-abdominal pressure (Fig. 9).

These products can have varying degrees of success that are dependent on the surgeon's experience and familiarity, and ultimately it is for each individual to find a method of fogging prevention best suited to his/her preference and style. Methods of fogging prevention are now seen as crucial for the smooth execution of laparoscopic surgery, and it is not uncommon to see multiple methods used in combination during the course of a single procedure.

Gas Insufflator

The insufflator is an essential element in laparoscopic surgery, which creates optimal operative space for facilitation of surgical procedures. It creates and maintains the pneumoperitoneum, and controls the intra-abdominal gas pressure during surgery.

An insufflator works as a pressure-controlled closed circuit, and gas is provided by a bottle with a pressure of 50–200 bars, or by a centrally

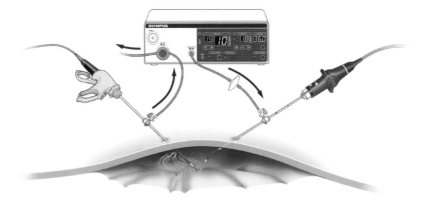

Figure 9. Illustration on how an active suction-insufflation device operates. (Copyright© 2014 Olympus. All rights reserved. Used with permission of Olympus.)

supplied wall unit (3.5–5 bars). A flow control valve regulates gas delivery and monitors the pressure in the circuit, allowing for different flow rates for insufflation. The insufflator can only accurately measure intra-abdominal pressure when there is minimal gas flow since at that moment, there is pressure equilibrium between the insufflator and the peritoneal cavity. For this reason, the insufflator creates the pneumoperitoneum in a rapid cyclical fashion. The total volume of gas delivered to the patient is measured, and in the presence of a major leak, this value will rise steeply — indicating that the gas bottle is being emptied rapidly. The usual maximum pressure allowed is in the region of 12 mm Hg, and many insufflators have mechanisms that prevent the accidental increase in pressure to more than 15 mm Hg (see Fig. 1). It is not uncommon however, for surgeons to increase the pressure deliberately under certain situations if they feel it will help facilitate the procedure.

An ideal insufflator is one that: (1) permits a high flow rate; (2) humidifies the gas; (3) displays pertinent values such as flow rate, volume, and pressure; and (4) is equipped with a pressure alarm and automatically exsufflates in situations of excessive pressure. Automatic exsufflation reduces the risk of gas embolism in cases of excessive pneumoperitoneum pressures. Humidifying the gas reduces the heat loss from patient during surgery, and should ideally be performed under sterile conditions. Carbon dioxide is gradually eliminated from the pneumoperitoneum during laparoscopic surgery due to its high diffusion capacity and excretion by respiration. It is replaced partially in the pneumoperitoneum by the anaesthetic gas nitrous oxide, and this increases the risk of gas embolism (due to nitrous oxide's poor solubility) and explosion (due to nitrous oxide's reactive nature). Continuous, automatic replacement of carbon dioxide by the insufflator to maintain an adequate level of carbon dioxide within the abdominal cavity mitigates these risks.

As mentioned previously, an automated suction-insufflator device allows gas to be aspirated from the operative field and to compensate the aspirated gas, volume for volume, with injected gas. The system aspirates the gas continuously and compensates for this loss by injecting new gas through a second port (Fig. 9). Certain insufflators warm the carbon dioxide gas before it enters the peritoneal cavity, its main aim being to prevent the cooling of the body, hence decreasing the metabolic and physiological issues associated with hypothermia.

Air, oxygen and nitrous oxide were initially experimented with for creation of the pneumoperitoneum, but fell out of favour for various reasons. Carbon dioxide is currently the standard gas used in modern laparoscopic surgery for its inert nature and rapid clearance by respiration when absorbed, thereby reducing the risk of gas embolism. Helium has had some success in endocrine surgery while xenon may offer some cardiac stability, but both are very rarely used.

Trocars and Instrument Ports

Trocars, with their sharp or blunt tips, allow for the insertion of instrument ports through the abdominal wall under direct vision. There is a great range of models to choose from commercially, but their basic shape and function remain the same (Figs. 10–13).

Plastic trocars and ports reduce the risk of thermal injury to the abdominal wall as compared to metal-based trocars and ports. However, they are

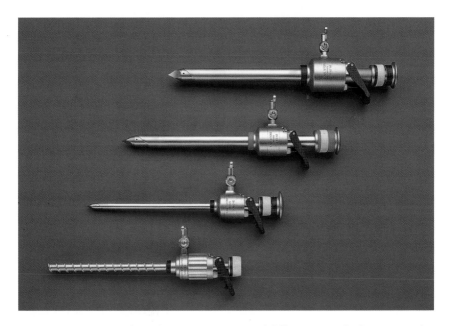

Figure 10. An array of metal trocar/port systems of different sizes, The bottom port has ridges, which allow for better traction against the abdominal wall to prevent displacement of the port intra-operatively, but may be more traumatic. These are re-usable. (Copyright© 2014 Karl Storz. All rights reserved. Used with permission of Karl Storz.)

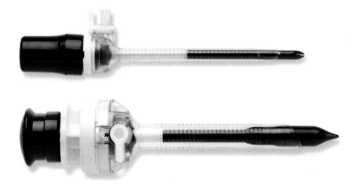

Figure 11.   Examples of non-reusable plastic trocar/port systems. These too have ridges, albeit less pronounced than the one depicted on the metal ports in Fig. 10. (Copyright© 2014 Covidien. All rights reserved. Used with permission of Covidien.)

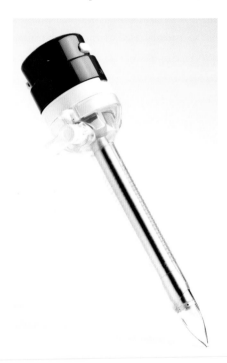

Figure 12.   An optical trocar/port system. A laparoscope can be placed within the trocar during insertion, with the trocar's clear, pointed tip allowing the surgeon to visualise the layers of the abdominal wall as the trocar is advanced. Once the peritoneal cavity is entered, the trocar is removed and the laparoscope re-inserted into the port. (Copyright© 2014 Covidien All rights reserved. Used with permission of Covidien.)

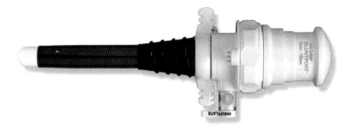

Figure 13. An example of a blunt port, used for the initial Hassan method cannulation. (Copyright© 2014 Covidien. All rights reserved. Used with permission of Covidien.)

non-reusable and significantly more expensive. There are specialised optical trocar/port systems which allows for a 0° laparoscope to be inserted into the wall within the trocar, enabling the surgeon to visualise when the trocar has entered the peritoneal cavity. The trocar tip may contain a spring-loaded mechanism and automatically retracts when reactionary forces from abdominal wall structures are lost upon entering the peritoneal cavity. This is most beneficial in morbidly obese patients where a conventional Hassan method of pneumoperitoneum creation is technically challenging.

The authors usually make use of one 10 mm Hassan port to be placed at the sub-umbilical region, and three 5 mm ports to be placed along the sub-xiphoid and right subcostal margin. Two of the 5 mm right subcostal ports can be exchanged for 3 mm sized ports in some instances. In patients with a thin abdominal wall undergoing an elective procedure, an even smaller port ("needlescope") measuring 1.7 mm can be utilised.

The authors routinely gain access to the abdomen via the open Hassan method, and do not make use of a Veress needle (Fig. 14). We believe this reduces the risk of inadvertent vascular and visceral injuries when creating the pneumoperitonuem. However, this may be an option in the morbidly obese where Hassan cannulation is difficult, and an optical trocar/port system is not readily available.

Electrocautery Equipment and Energy Devices

An ideal electrosurgical device offers consistency, utility, reliability, efficiency and safety. The choice of device used in any particular surgery depends greatly on local expertise, product availability and economy.

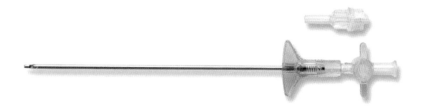

Figure 14.   A Veress needle system. (Copyright© 2014 Covidien. All rights reserved. Used with permission of Covidien.)

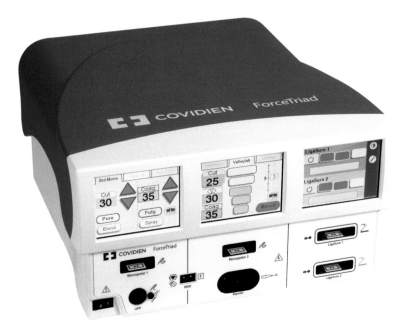

Figure 15.   ForceTriad™, a commonly used electrocautery energy source. It allows for multiple electrocautery modalities to be utilised concurrently. (Copyright© 2014 Covidien. All rights reserved. Used with permission of Covidien.)

Of all the modern energy equipment available, monopolar cautery remains the most widely used during laparoscopic cholecystectomy. There are two modes of monopolar cautery, coagulation and cutting, with coagulation mode being used almost exclusively during laparoscopy. Electrical energy from an energy generator (Fig. 15) is dispersed from the active smaller electrode on the laparoscopic instrument to a larger return electrode, the grounding pad (commonly placed in the buttocks or thighs). Concentration of current at the smaller electrode allows for haemostatic cutting and coagulation.

However, injuries are common with monopolar cautery for a variety of reasons. The instrument shaft has current passing through it and if the insulation of the shaft is damaged, direct coupling can injure tissues touching the shaft. Inorganic objects such as the laparoscope, instruments, or clips may be energised and result in indirect damage to tissues. Capacitive coupling can also occur when current is transferred from the active electrode through the intact insulation into adjacent materials without direct contact due to potential differences between the two conductors.

Bipolar diathermy technology combines an active electrode and a return electrode into a single electrosurgical instrument with two small poles. Rather than passing through the patient from the active electrode to the grounding pad, the alternating current is distributed through the target tissue. Lower voltages are needed to achieve the same tissue effect in bipolar electrosurgery as those achieved in monopolar because the poles are closer to each other. Bipolar electrosurgery thus results in less potential damage to surrounding tissues and less risk of capacitive coupling. Bipolar forceps allow for firm grasping and reliable coagulation of vessels less than 3 mm in size.

A few commercially available bipolar and ultrasonic instruments have been developed, including Ligasure™, Enseal™, Harmonic™, Thunderbeat™, Caiman™, Gyrus™. Locally, Ligasure™, Harmonic™, Enseal™ and

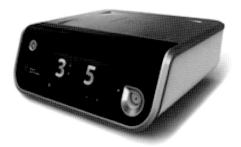

Figure 16. Ethicon Endo-Surgery™ generator that is commonly used together with the Harmonic™ (see below) energy device (Copyright© 2014 Ethicon. All rights reserved. Used with permission of Ethicon.)

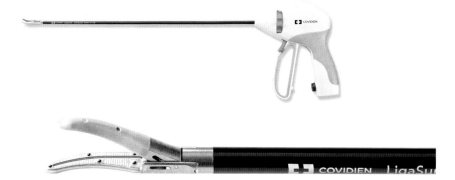

Figure 17. The Maryland tip version of Ligasure™. (Copyright© 2014 Covidien. All rights reserved. Used with permission of Covidien.)

Thunderbeat™ are the most commonly available. Sonicision™, an industry-first cordless ultrasonic device, has also been recently introduced.

The Ligasure™ device delivers high current, low voltage along with pressure from the jaws to tissue. The instrument can seal vessels up to 7 mm in size. This is in contrast to the high voltage, low current energy used in standard monopolar and bipolar cautery. The system monitors the energy expended and during the cooling phase of the cycle, cross-linking of the denatured collagen and elastin re-occurs creating a new seal. The instrument is available in 5 or 10 mm sizes. Tissue sensing technology in the Ligasure™ makes use of a computer algorithm to adjust the current and voltage based on real-time measurements of tissue impedance, resulting in a constant delivery of wattage over a broad range of tissue types. It is usually used in conjunction with the ForceTriad™ energy generator (Figs. 15 and 17).

The Harmonic™ is a high frequency ultrasonic transducer. The active titanium blade vibrates at 55,000 cycles per second, and the resulting mechanical energy causes a breakdown of protein in tissues, which creates a coagulum. Vessel and tissue sealing is dependent on the power setting as well as the pressure exerted, the formation of the coagulum and tissue tension. The surgeon, permitting different tissue effects, can adjust the variability of energy delivered. The Harmonic™ performs at lower temperatures (50–100°C) than other devices (150–400°C), hence decreasing the collateral desiccation and charring. The active blade of the Harmonic™ can also be used as a knife. Available 5 mm blades include hook, straight and curved electrodes. Curved

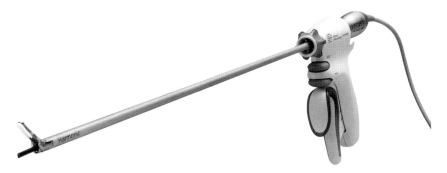

Figure 18. A version of the Harmonic™ ultrasonic energy device. (Copyright© 2014 Ethicon. All rights reserved. Used with permission of Ethicon.)

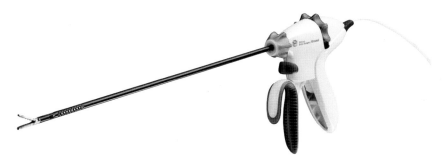

Figure 19. A laparoscopic version of Enseal™. (Copyright© 2014 Ethicon. All rights reserved. Used with permission of Ethicon.)

blades are more versatile and allow for work around difficult anatomical angles; as the blade is able to follow the direction of tissue, the rate of tissue transaction is faster. However, haemostasis is superior with the straight blade. The Harmonic™ is able to seal vessels up to 5 mm. It is used in conjunction with the Ethicon Endo-Surgery™ generator (Figs. 16 and 18).

The Enseal™ can seal and cut up to 7 mm vessels and lymphatics consistently through high uniform compression. It claims to have more consistent seal strength over multiple activations as compared with its competitors. It is versatile as well, being able to deliver energy to tissue even with the jaws open. Its technology allows it to maintain a tissue temperature of approximately 100°C, minimising tissue sticking, charring and smoke, as well as reducing thermal spread of energy to adjacent tissues. In addition, it comes in an articulating version, which allows easier access in tighter spots.

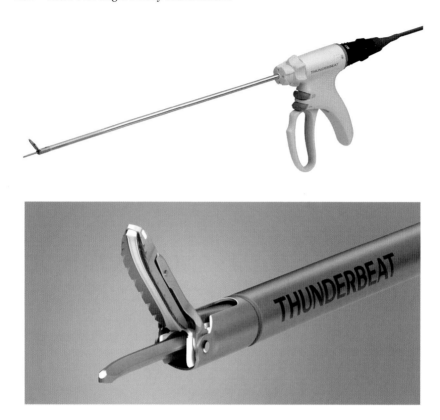

Figure 20. The Thunderbeat™. (Copyright© 2014 Olympus. All rights reserved. Used with permission of Olympus.)

Thunderbeat™ is a relatively new electrosurgical device that offers integration of advanced bipolar and ultrasonic energy, allowing the simultaneous actions of cutting and sealing. It boasts precise dissection with fine jaws, and minimal thermal spread. It has less mist generation, cuts tissue faster when compared to other advanced energy devices and can seal vessels up to 7 mm.

First of its kind in the market, the Sonicision™ is a cordless ultrasonic device that reliably seal vessels up to 5 mm in diameter. It claims to have less thermal spread, faster dissection speeds, less plume production, and a faster active blade cool-down time compared to its rivals. However, its greatest advantage is probably that of its cordless convenience and reusable battery.

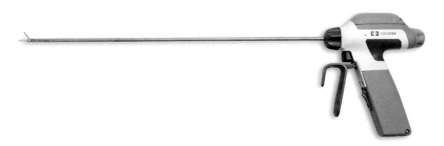

Figure 21. The Sonicision™. (Copyright© 2014 Covidien. All rights reserved. Used with permission of Covidien.)

Plasma consists of ionised gas in the form of high-energy particles. When enough heat is applied to argon gas, the electrons and argon ions separate to form pure argon plasma. Argon plasma coagulation (APC) involves the use of a jet of plasma that is directed through a probe which is passed through the endoscope. The probe is placed at some distance from the bleeding lesion, and argon gas is emitted and ionised by a high voltage discharge. High-frequency electrical current is then conducted through the jet of gas, resulting in coagulation of the bleeding lesion on the other end of the jet.

In reality however, most surgeons stick to monopolar instruments as their main source of electrocautery during laparoscopic cholecystectomy, saving the use of these complex and often expensive equipment for more complex surgical procedures. Different procedures may call for the use of different energy sealing devices, even the use of more than one in a procedure — depending on the type of dissection required by the surgeon.

Laparoscopic Instruments

There are a wide variety of laparoscopic instruments available for the grasping, dissecting, clipping, and cutting of tissues (Figs. 22–24).

Some of the more commonly used ones are Maryland curved dissectors, "dolphin-nosed" forceps, Reddick forceps, scissors, straight or curved bowel forceps, L-hook, and spatula. Each of these instruments has a role to play, and it is up to the surgeon's discretion on when and how each instrument is used. The authors prefer to use the Reddick forceps for grasping and retraction of the gallbladder, the dolphin-nosed forceps for precise electrocautery

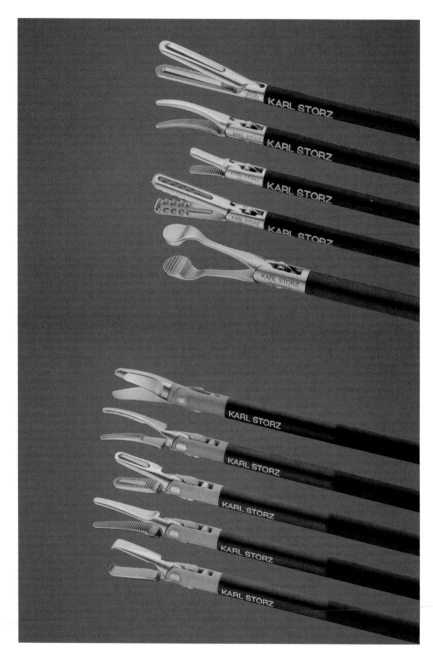

Figure 22.   Some examples of commonly used laparoscopic instruments. (Copyright© 2014 Karl Storz. All rights reserved. Used with permission of Karl Storz.)

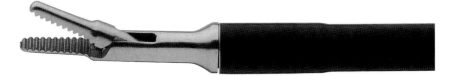

Figure 23. The dolphin-nosed forceps is an author's favourite for precise dissection. (Copyright© 2014 Karl Storz. All rights reserved. Used with permission of Karl Storz.)

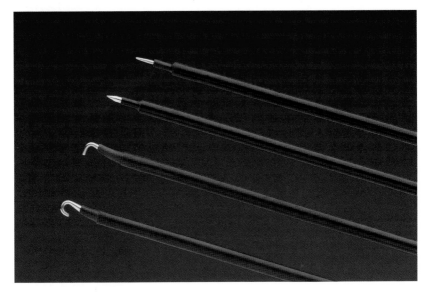

Figure 24. A selection of different hooks and tips for pinpoint dissection. (Copyright© 2014 Karl Storz. All rights reserved. Used with permission of Karl Storz.)

dissection of Calot's triangle, and the L-hook for the dissection of the gallbladder off the liver.

The laparoscopic suction irrigator is a special instrument, which allows for suction and irrigation to be applied via the same apparatus, with an inlet connected to a sterile water source, and an outlet connected to a vacuum (Fig. 25). Irrigation helps in blunt dissection, and dilutes peritoneal contamination in cases of bile spillage or severe inflammation.

A laparoscopic clip applicator is commonly used for the clipping of the cystic artery and duct (Fig. 26). Many different models, including re-usable or disposable types are routinely employed but their primary aim remains the

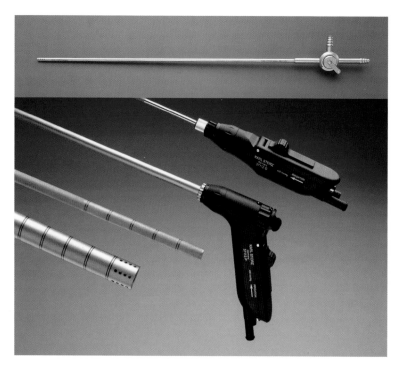

Figure 25. Different suction irrigators. (Copyright© 2014 Karl Storz. All rights reserved. Used with permission of Karl Storz.)

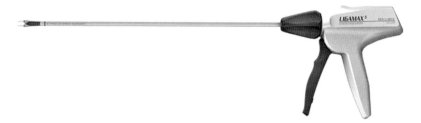

Figure 26. The Ligamax™, a commonly used laparoscopic clip applicator. (Copyright© 2014 Ethicon. All rights reserved. Used with permission of Ethicon.)

same. In cases in which oedema or chronic distension of the cystic duct causes its size to preclude clipping by a clip applicator, sutures may be needed to ligate the cystic duct via an intracorporeal or extracorporeal method. Laparoscopic vascular staplers have also been used to ligate the cystic duct and artery in cases where oedema and fibrosis prevent the use of clips.

Extra-long laparoscopic instruments are available for use in obese patients whose thicker abdominal walls make it difficult for standard length instruments to reach the intended operative field.

Gauze Strips

The authors routinely use gauze strips in their laparoscopic cholecystectomies, with the severity and complexity of the case dictating the number of gauze strips used. These gauze strips are about 5 cm in length, each with their own radio-opaque identifiers (Fig. 27).

It is very useful as a blunt dissector when held with a grasper and manipulated in a circular or up-down motion. As an absorbent material for the blood and liquid fat from the dissection process, it aids greatly in keeping the visual field relatively clean and dry, and thus the optical images clear and crisp. Lastly, its white colour provides contrast against the tissues for better anatomical visualisation and recognition by the surgeon. They are easily inserted via the 10 mm Hassan port, and can be removed together with the gallbladder in a laparoscopic retrieval device. We commonly employ at least three of these gauze strips in simple elective cases, with more inserted as required.

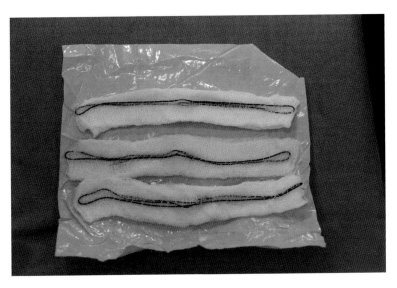

Figure 27. Gauze strips favoured by the authors during laparoscopic cholecystectomy.

Fears that excessive use of gauze strips may lead to missing pieces intra-operatively are largely unfounded, especially since the operative field is limited to the upper right quadrant. Careful accounting of all gauze strips by the surgical team and awareness by the surgeon of where he/she has placed the gauze strips can eliminate this potential complication.

Drains

Drains are not routinely used by the authors, but can be useful in cases where massive bile spillage and contamination has occurred. It allows for the continued drainage of fluid and stale blood from the subphrenic and subhepatic spaces to prevent a potential collection or abscess formation. They also serve to indicate a bile leak for early intervention. The drains used are usually plastic, small calibre and connected to active suction provided by vacuum-sealed bottles. They are removed at the surgeon's clinical discretion and judgment, usually 1–3 days post-operatively.

Retrieval Devices

A range of laparoscopic specimen retrieval devices exists in the market specially designed to allow for the easy retrieval of organs and other equipment from the abdominal cavity after surgery is completed. These are usually inserted through the 10 mm periumbilical port towards the end of surgery. They are usually made of tough, plastic material that can withstand a certain amount of pulling force. They have built-in deployment and closure systems that utilise a push-pull motion and are generally easy to use. A laparoscope (either a 10 mm or 5 mm sized one) is usually inserted via the epigastric port during this part of the procedure to allow for retrieval of the specimen and gauze strips under direct vision. The retrieval device with its contents is then pulled back out through the periumbilical port at the end of the procedure.

The authors currently prefer to use a simple disposable plastic pouch with a purse-string suture and sliding knot incorporated at its opening. The pouch is inserted via the 10 mm periumbilical port, with the end of the suture remaining outside the body. The bag is positioned above the liver surface and the gallbladder with gauze strips placed inside, before simultaneously holding onto the sliding knot and pulling on the suture outside the

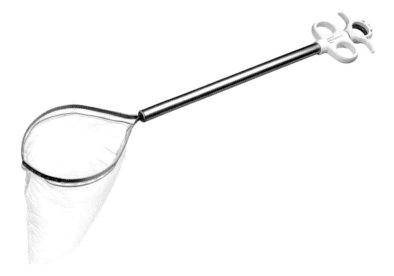

Figure 28. The Endo-Catch™, a commonly used specimen retrieval pouch readily available. (Copyright© 2014 Covidien. All rights reserved. Used with permission of Covidien.)

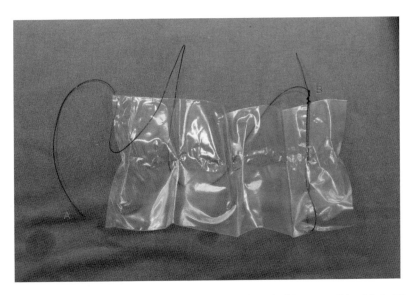

Figure 29. The plastic pouch is closed by pulling on the end of the suture (A), while holding onto the sliding knot (B).

body to close the pouch. This has the advantage of allowing the laparoscope to remain inserted via the periumbilical port for the entirety of the operation. As such, this avoids the switching of laparoscopes or adjustments to a relatively unfamiliar view. The pouch is then removed via the periumbilical incision at the end of surgery.

Index

accessory ducts of Luschka, 5
acute cholecystitis, 35
acute myocardial ischaemia, 91
acute pancreatitis, 39
adhesiolysis, 128
adhesions, 128, 129, 131
ampulla of Vater, 3, 30, 47
amylase, 39
anti-coagulants, 53
anti-fog solutions, 151
anti-platelets, 53
aorta, 92
argon plasma coagulation, 163
ascites, 119
atelactasis, 91

bile, 3, 5, 6, 11
bile ducts, 3
bile salts, 6, 7, 11
bile spillage, 120
biliary colic, 18, 20, 26, 35
biliary-enteric fistula, 40

bilirubin, 12
bipolar diathermy, 159

calcium, 12
calcium bilirubinate, 12
calculous cholecystitis, 20
Calot's triangle, 6, 66, 67, 69, 92, 125, 128
Camper's fascia, 59
cardiovascular, 51, 52
central computing unit, 149
cerebrovascular accident, 91, 118
Charcot's triad, 36
chlorhexidine, 53
cholangiopancreatography, 45
cholangitis, 25, 26, 36, 39, 40
cholecystectomy, 1, 17
cholecystitis, 21, 23
cholecysto-colonic fistula, 133
cholecysto-enteric fistulas, 132
choledocholithiasis, 25, 36, 38
cholesterol gallstone, 12, 15

cholesterol stones, 15
chronic cholecystitis, 25, 40
cirrhosis, 31
Cloquet's node, 69, 125
coagulopathy, 32
common bile duct, 3, 25–27, 42
common bile duct injury, 93
complications, 91
computer tomography, 43
Cullen's sign, 37
cystic artery, 5, 6, 88
cystic duct, 3–6, 18, 35

3D, 143
da vinci, 115
deep vein thrombosis, 91
drains, 88, 122, 168
duodenum, 3, 7

empyema, 23, 35, 124
endoscopic retrograde
    cholangiopancreatography
    (ERCP), 27, 29, 31, 47
endoscopic ultrasound, 42
Enseal, 159, 161

falciform ligament, 88, 119
fatty liver, 38
ForceTriad, 160

gallbladder, 3–5, 7
gallbladder cancer, 32, 33
gallbladder carcinoma, 122
gallbladder polyp, 17
gallstone, 11, 12, 35
gangrenous cholecystitis, 23, 24, 124
gas insufflator, 153

gauze strips, 167
Grey-Turner's sign, 37

haemorrhage, 88, 118
Harmonic, 159–161
Hartmann's pouch, 4, 30
Hassan, 62, 66, 91, 131, 157
hepatic artery, 3
hepatic duct, 3
hernia, 88, 119, 138
high-definition, 147

ileus, 88, 99
incisional hernia, 88, 111, 124
intra-abdominal collection, 120
irrigation, 77, 81, 121
ischaemic heart disease, 118

jaundice, 36

Kocher's (subcostal) incision, 56, 88

laparoscope, 145, 146
laparoscope warmers, 151
laparoscopic cholecystectomy, 1, 2, 27, 29, 51, 135, 136
laparoscopic ultrasound, 43
laparoscopy, 1
Ligasure, 159, 160
lipase, 39
liver, 3
liver cirrhosis, 118
lymph node of Cloquet, 6

magnetic resonance imaging, 45
metabolic syndrome, 118
Mirizzi's syndrome, 30, 31
mixed gallstones, 15

monopolar cautery, 158
Morrison's pouch, 78, 97
mucocele, 35
Murphy's sign, 21, 35, 40

necrotising fasciitis, 97
needlescopic, 84, 85

obese, 117
open cholecystectomy, 136

pancreatic duct, 3
pancreatitis, 30, 36, 39
percutaneous cholecystotomy, 24
perforation, 95, 124
peripheral vascular disease, 118
peritonitis, 24
pigment gallstone, 12
pneumonia, 91
pneumoperitoneum, 52
porcelain (calcified) gallbladder, 17,
    40, 122
portal hypertension, 88, 119
portal vein, 3
post-cholecystectomy syndrome, 101
pregnancy, 31
pregnant, 31
pseudo-triangulation, 111
pulmonary, 52
pulmonary embolism, 91

rectus sheath, 60, 61
renal failure, 52
renal impairment, 118
retrieval devices, 74, 76, 168
Reynold's pentad, 36
right hepatic artery, 88
right paracolic gutter, 78
robotics, 143
robotic surgery, 115, 116

Scarpa's fascia, 59
scintigraphy, 49
single incision, 107
sphincter of Oddi, 3, 101
subphrenic, 78
subtotal cholecystectomy, 126

third dimensional space, 105
three-dimensional, 103
thrombosis, 52
Thunderbeat, 159, 160, 162
transabdominal ultrasound, 40
transient ischaemic attack, 91

vena cava, 92
Veress, 91, 131

wound infection, 81, 87, 96, 97, 138